NO EXCUSES!

The "War On Obesity"

A stern, non-"politically correct" view of our nations Overly Fat People

---

Rick Bobzien

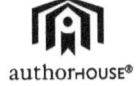

authorHOUSE®

AuthorHouse™
1663 Liberty Drive
Bloomington, IN 47403
www.authorhouse.com
Phone: 1-800-839-8640

First published by AuthorHouse 2/25/2010

ISBN: 978-1-4490-7895-9 (e)
ISBN: 978-1-4490-7897-3 (sc)
ISBN: 978-1-4490-7896-6 (hc)

Library of Congress Control Number: 2010901712

Printed in the United States of America
Bloomington, Indiana

This book is printed on acid-free paper.

TABLE OF CONTENTS

Preface   **ix**

FROM DENIAL TO ACCEPTANCE AND ACCOUNTABILITY

Chapter One: Definition of an Overly Fat Person   **1**
  Methods and techniques for diagnosis

Chapter Two: Character and Personality   **11**
  It is you! Accountability for one's actions

RATIONALIZATIONS AND CONTRIBUTING FACTORS

Chapter Three: Genetics   **21**
  Disproving the genetics rationalization. Proving
  accountability

Chapter Four: Societal Influences   **29**
  Attitudes - empathy, "Big and Beautiful" & "Full Figured"
  to television, etc

Chapter Five: Pregnancy   **41**
  A common rationalization by women for their obesity

Chapter Six: I am a Man!   49
    How perceived "machismo" contributes to the obesity problem

Chapter Seven: Sports   55
    How professional sports are influential and insightful

REASONS TO LOSE THE WEIGHT

Chapter Eight: Physical Health   63
    Health issues with respect to obesity

Chapter Nine: Mental Health   73
    How being "normal" can improve one's mental outlook

Chapter Ten: Additional Advantages to Losing Weight   79
    Reasons every "Overly Fat Person" should lose weight

Chapter Eleven: Pollution   91
    How obese people negatively affect others

REMEDIES FOR THE OBESITY EPIDEMIC

Chapter Twelve: Diets And Weight Loss   97
    Do diets work? - Save money! - Some useful advice

Chapter Thirteen: The Competitiveness Factor   115
    Pro's and con's to competitiveness and how to best utilize your personality

Chapter Fourteen: Societal Actions   129
    How society should fight the nations obesity epidemic

THE NEGATIVE RESPONSE TO THIS BOOK!

Chapter Fifteen: The Outcry   **137**
    From "Fat Sympathizers" to entities that will lose revenues

Conclusion   **151**

PREFACE

Warning! This book is not for the faint at heart. This book is
reality. And reality can be brutally painful.

Read on if you dare!

IF YOU ARE LIKE MANY AMERICANS, you are FAT. You're not
"pudgy." You're not "husky." You're not "Full Figured." You're not a
"Large Person." You're just plain and simply FAT! You're probably
what most of the other civilized world considers a "Fat American
Pig." What you really are is an "Overly Fat Person" who is "Fat And
Totally Accountable." For the remainder of this book I will use the
acronym OFP for an "Overly Fat Person."

The main purpose of this book is to reveal the true reasons for
Americans being so fat. Americans are fat for basically a few simple
reasons. One, they lack any self-control or discipline with respect
to food and drink. Two, they are lazy. Three, they are apathetic;
they don't care about or respect their body; basically they "don't give
a damn." And because of our society's attitude toward being fat is
becoming more tolerant, it is totally acceptable for people to remain
in this repulsive condition of obesity; so they do. And as common
sense dictates, any combination of the before mentioned, cause
people to become OFP's.

It is also the premise of this author that being an Overly Fat Person is a personality/character trait. Thus, this repulsive and despicable condition of being an OFP can be prevented and or altered if so desired. Thus, there is no excuse for individuals to allow themselves to become obese. This lack of initiative toward maintaining one's body in a healthy and dignified state shows other people that an "Overly Fat Person" does not care about their body. It is similar to a person not bathing or washing ones hair for a week or more. It's the same thing as if a person doesn't take the time to brush his or her teeth for a year. And when one thinks about the health problems fat people face for remaining in this disgusting condition of obesity, it is as if an obese person is playing Russian roulette.

And if it is not obvious already, it is the premise of the author that being fat is disgusting. And the more an individual is overweight the more disgusting the condition. It is "Visual Pollution." It is repulsive! The author believes that people can do something about their disgusting condition and when they don't they are a disgusting person…. Or, should I say, an OFP. They, OFP's may be nice people, but people who commit crimes are sometimes nice people too. Criminals probably have friends and co-workers who consider them to be nice. Nice has nothing to do with it! Yes, you can be nice and be severely overweight. You would then be a nice, overweight and depending on the severity of the person's obesity, a disgusting person.

Of course there is more to this book then just letting people know that they're fat; or that a good portion of our population is fat. Or of telling fat people how to lose weight. This book will also give tips on how to become… not skinny, not slim, but "NORMAL." Yes, normal! Well, a better term would be natural. It is not natural to be fat (And don't give me any of that survival storing of fat excuse). It might become "normal" if trends in the U.S. continue but it is not natural. It is obvious to the author that "normal" in America is now very close to being fat. But it is not normal around the world. And there is no reason it should be normal and natural here in the United States.

This book will show you how (sorry, it can't do it for you) that by changing your attitude and your lifestyle that it is possible to rid yourself of that disgusting fat. This book will be beneficial for the reader in many different ways. There are chapters in this book on determining if you are an Overly Fat Person. There are chapters in this book on diets and diet fads and what a waste of money (for you, not for those making money off you) these diets can be. There are also chapters on exercise and like diets, the fads, the fact, fiction and rampant propaganda. There are sections in this book on the benefits of not being an "Overly Fat Person." Benefits of not being an "Overly Fat Person" range from an individuals general health to the fact that being in shape makes a person more attractive to the opposite sex. There are chapters on attitudes…. especially in today's American society. There is a chapter on competitiveness and the pros and cons for individuals trying to maintain a healthy weight or lose unwanted weight. There is also a chapter on genetics and how minimal the role of genetics is in relation to obesity. Everything you really need to know about being fat or how to avoid being an "Overly Fat Person" or how to get back to a natural healthy weight if you are an "OFP" are included in this book. And more!

It also bears mentioning that this book will be met with much criticism. It is extremely important that this be mentioned! Any book that actually points out the facts and dispels many, many misleading theories and so-called facts will be met with harsh criticism and skepticism. And of course, heaven forbid if someone is not politically correct! And any book that can save people money while simultaneously taking money from others and consequently, those entities losing revenue, will rebel against this book. In short, this book threatens many!

This book, if taken to heart, will change your life and the lives of others. But the decision is yours! Read on if you have the courage. Read on if you wish to change your life or help our society rid itself of the cancer of the fat epidemic, of the Overly Fat People. Or, just close the book, laugh or mumble an obscenity and let yourself and our country continue the downward spiral. Or worse yet, if you are an Overly Fat Person……… close the book and remain fat!

Chapter One

DEFINITION OF AN OVERLY FAT PERSON

So, YOU HAVE DECIDED TO READ further. Maybe this is due to your curiosity. Maybe you are already disgusted with the author and you want to read further to build up your animosity and also gain ammunition to further critique the outlandish (obviously your opinion not mine) claims that people can actually control their bodies through some form of accountability. Or, maybe you are a fat person who needs some form of self-help, some prodding which would enable you to lose weight and thus lead a more normal life. If so, congratulations! But, for whatever reason you are continuing to read further, to fully understand the book you must have a definition of an Overly Fat Person.

Having a definition is also important because many individuals, who are indeed fat, don't consider themselves fat. It totally amazes me about what is occurring in our society these days. In our society today many, many people who are overly fat actual think they are just fine with respect to their body weight. Much of these feelings of contentment by overweight and obese individuals stems from denial. And unfortunately this comes with full support and empathy from large portions of our society. Some of this denial by fat people also

1

comes from the fact that they feel somewhat normal because so many in our society are overweight. An overweight person is conditioned to feel normal and feels totally comfortable with themselves because they "fit in." There will be more on these thoughts in later chapters.

So what classifies a person as an OFP? Are we talking about what the medical community classifies as "Morbidly Obese?" Are we considering people who are "Obese" as being an Overly Fat Person? Or are we labeling individuals who fall under the medical communities classification of "Overweight" as being OFP's?

I have actually given this much thought, this need to easily determine a method to classify an individual as an OFP. At first, I thought of defining the OFP condition by considering anyone more than 10-15 pounds heavier then the normal healthy individuals body weight as an OFP. But this posed obvious problems. First, what is the definition of a "Normal" person and whose definition would be the most accurate. And the second problem posed by using "normal" body weight as the standard, is that what was normal in the 1960's for example, is not what would be considered normal in today's society.

Another issue with using "Normal" as a base to determine if someone is an OFP is that "Normal" is often considered as what is "Average" amongst the population. So, if that is the case, then we have even more problems. We then have problems such as which population should be considered, the United States population? Boy, wouldn't that make it easy for all the fat people, seeing as to how the average person in the United States now is probably medically considered "Overweight." Gee, let's add 10 to 15 pounds to an individual's weight who is already overweight to determine an Overly Fat Person's weight. Or maybe the world's population should be used to determine a standard? Or how about the population of Japan? No, "Normal" or "Average" is not a great method to determine if an individual is an OFP.

I also considered the various medical communities height and weight charts with all the different scales/variables for men, women, children, and various ages, bone structures, etc. Yikes!!!!!!!

No, that would not be a great method of determination. Besides, some in the medical community actually think just because we reach middle age or older that we should naturally become heavier. Some in the medical community must feel that an individual is not capable of adjusting their caloric intake as their metabolisms or daily activity levels change. That way of thought is part of our cultures philosophy that contributes to Overly Fat People and our nations fat epidemic; so why on earth would I deem these medical charts and scales a great yardstick?

And yes, I even thought of the BMI (Body Mass Index) garbage that is out there for all of us to ponder. Take it from someone who works out, the BMI index is a piece of garbage. It is amazing, and actually alarming (we sometimes trust them, don't we?) that the scientific community could come up with something with so many obvious shortcomings. You take any male or female athlete or even an everyday individual who lifts any weights what so ever and it throws the BMI completely off. Forget the BMI! Forget the height and weight charts!

Years ago, like in the 70's or 80's, if I had been asked the question of what is overweight and how I would classify someone as an Overly Fat Person I would have given definite consideration to a persons waistline when graduating from High School. But like all segments of our nations population the increase in obesity amongst high school students/graduates has increased significantly. Drive by any high school when the students are walking about and take a look at their bodies. It is a sad observation indeed! What you will see is a large percentage of the students being overweight. And large percentages, even though only high school aged, are OFP's at 18 years of age or younger. This is so sad and begs you to ask what these kids parents are thinking (the parents are probably fat too!) and how much do these kids actually consume on a daily basis. Considering a teenager's metabolism, it is not easy to be a fat teenager; they have to work at it. And of course the sad and scarier thought is what are these individuals going to look like at 30 or 40 years of age if they don't change their lifestyles? What are these fat individuals' chances of leading a healthy life if they continue down the destructive path of obesity? Well, if they continue down the obesity path their future is pretty bleak and extremely sad, that's all I can say!

So how in the world do I define being an Overly Fat Person? What measuring device, what standard do I use and justify? There are a few methods but all relate to one methodology, Visual. Yes, I know, how subjective can you be? But not really! If an individual is brutally honest with themselves then a good look in the mirror or a critical look at some photographs will do the trick and determine for a person if indeed they are entering or have entered the realm of the OFP's. And this look/analysis needs to be done with as little clothes on as possible, preferably a view of an individual's naked body. Many fashions these days are very clever about concealing a person's shortcomings, especially with respect to body weight. And yes, if you are too embarrassed about your body to look in the mirror or have a photo taken of you then you are more then likely an OFP; or so shy that maybe you need some psychiatric help.

So what does a person analyze when looking at oneself in the mirror or a photograph? How can someone be objective with respect to whether or not they are an Overly Fat Person? It's pretty simple, if you see rolls of fat on your body then duh, you're a fat person. If you turn sideways and look in a mirror and your gut is sticking out then you are a fat person. If you face a mirror and if you suck in your gut and tighten your muscles and you don't look like a model that is relaxed then you are probably an OFP or getting extremely close.

If you have more than just a little fat hanging over your pants then you are an Overly Fat Person. If when you are sitting down on the toilet and you look down at your belly… if it is large then guess what? Yes, you are an OFP. And we won't even go there with respect to if you can see your genitals when sitting on the toilet.

Another visual method to determine if you are an "Overly Fat Person" is the "book" method. This method has been around for years and I feel it is fairly accurate. The "book" method entails lying flat on your back on the floor and placing a large book on your stomach. If the book face tilts back toward your face you are overweight! However, this method has some obvious shortcomings. For instance, you can have monster thighs and huge love handles but if your abdomen is not very protruding the "book" method comes up short.

So what it basically boils down to is this; if an individual is more than about 15 to 20 pounds overweight then you will more than likely not look good in the mirror. This poor appearance, with a large protruding belly or rolls of fat makes you are an Overly Fat Person. Looking "good" in the mirror or in a photo is "NORMAL." This, "looking good is normal," is an extremely important concept for all of our society to understand and it will be reiterated throughout this book; that looking good in a photo or in the mirror… looking "hot" looking "sexy" is NORMAL. If a person is just 10-15 lbs from looking "Good" then they are NOT quite an OFP yet but without some caution they too will fall into the repulsive category and join our societies growing community of OFP.

But the point to remember is:

Looking "Good" is "Normal."

DON'T LET IT HAPPEN TO YOU!

THERE IS ONE LAST ITEM I would like to mention before moving on to other chapters. Many people don't realize how extremely easy it is to put on some extra pounds and how over the years those few extra pounds accumulate to the extent that a person can go from just a few pounds overweight to obese. If one considers what happens over a period of just one year if a person were to gain just one pound per month it is actually a very frightening thought. 12 pounds a year can quickly make a person obese, and that is pretty obvious. But what is less obvious is that 12 pounds a year is only a quarter pound of weight gain per week (I know, there are 52 weeks in a year which changes calculations slightly… give me a break!)! Even if an individual only puts on a couple of pounds a year this extra weight over the years can easily cause obesity. Think of a person 20 years old that gains 2 extra pounds a year. What will this person look and feel like when they are 40? And worse yet, it is more difficult to lose the weight as a person ages! So think about that the next time you have that extra piece of birthday cake or drink those 6 beers after dinner.

IF YOU ARE FAT...

YOU ARE NOT:

"AT RISK"

YOU ARE NOT:

"BIG AND BEAUTIFUL"

YOU ARE NOT:

"PLUMP"

YOU ARE FAT!

GET A LIFE! LOSE THE BAGGAGE!

REMEMBER!!!!!!! IF YOU ARE FAT IT IS BECAUSE OF ONE OR MORE OF THE FOLLOWING:

You are lazy and inactive

You lack any discipline or self-control with respect to food and drink

You are apathetic with respect to your physical condition…. You don't give a damn.

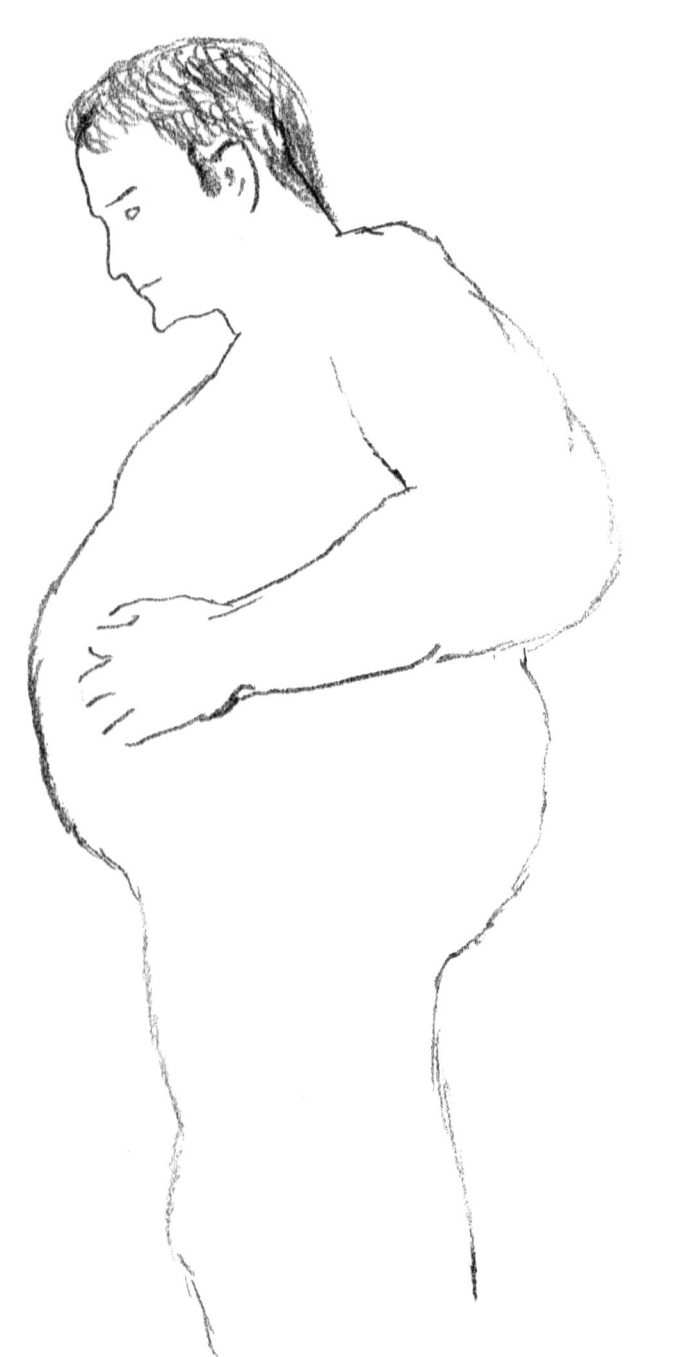

Chapter Two

CHARACTER AND PERSONALITY

THE MAJOR PREMISE OF THIS BOOK is that being obese, or an "Overly Fat Person" is a significant indicator of one's personality and character and that obese people should be treated as such. A fat persons disgusting condition of obesity is indeed part of their make-up/personality and they should be held accountable for their actions. If an individual has accountability for their actions it changes significantly how we should treat and perceive them. This accountability changes how we view fat people as individuals and whether or not and to what degree to respect them. And, on a more positive note, when "Overly Obese Individuals" begin to realize that they are being held accountable for their actions by the rest of society then their behaviors may change for the better.

This premise of an individual being overweight and that this individuals being overweight is basically their decision is of vital importance. It is vitally important because all the people who believe it is being too harsh to criticize individuals for being overweight typically believe that the obesity of an individual is to a very large degree, uncontrollable by the overweight person. These "Fat Sympathizers;" these people who think everything is a disease

11

or some uncontrollable mental or physical condition, think that someone who is obese has as much control over their weight as they do over their facial features! This is BULL!

Remember, as I indicated in the Forward, if you are fat it is because you are either:

Lazy, which leads to inactivity

Lacking in self-discipline and or self-control with respect to food and drink

Apathetic- Just not caring …lacking dignity and self-respect in regard to your body's appearance, health, etc.

LAZINESS

LET'S TAKE A LOOK AT THESE traits one at a time. First, let's look at laziness. Laziness is defined as "Disposed to be idle." That says a lot with respect to fat people, doesn't it?

Laziness is evil in two respects. First, if a person is lazy, they are lying around doing little to nothing. If a person is doing little to nothing they obviously are not burning much in the way of calories. So a lazy person is not jogging, going for walks, weightlifting, doing yard work, chores around the house, or other activities that not only burn calories when a person is active but also can actually raise an individuals metabolism for extended periods of time. Thus, this raising of metabolism is burning calories faster then normal even after the activity ceases. If an individual is extremely lazy none of these beneficial weight reducers are occurring.

If you disagree with this notion that many fat individuals are indeed fat because they are inactive, think about how often you see fat people jogging, playing soccer or tennis or engaged in physical activities. And I might mention that some of this lack of participation in physical activities is related to the embarrassment factor in which a fat person feels very embarrassed or too self-conscious to participate in many physically activities. This becomes a catch-22 for many Overly Fat People. Fat people are sometimes too self-conscious to be active and yet not being active contributes to their condition of obesity.

Now, here is an item of extreme importance regarding my attitude toward Overly Fat People. This item is not related to personality but interjecting this thought now before I am totally disrespected seems appropriate. Throughout this book I basically ridicule, condemn and insult overweight people for their condition of obesity because it is within their control to not be obese. But there is one scenario with respect to obese people of which I will not criticize or ridicule. And that scenario is when Overly Fat People are engaged in a physical activity and are thus DOING SOMETHING about their condition. In fact, I respect and applaud any overweight person who is working out and of course cutting down on their caloric intake. When I see an Overly Fat Person jogging down the street I think to myself "that takes guts." No, seriously, I realize how difficult it is for fat people to not only overcome the worry of what others are thinking about their bodies when jogging or swimming or whatever; but I realize that depending on a persons state of obesity, their degree of effort is substantially more than a fit individuals degree of effort for the same activity. **So I tremendously respect these individuals who are attempting to remedy their obesity condition!!!**

The second reason being lazy is evil, and this reason is probably just as sinister as the first reason, is that while you are lying around being lazy, you are very likely to be consuming calories. And, if this is in addition to an individuals normal 3 meals a day, well then there is an extreme likelihood that these extra calories will result in the accumulation of additional fat stores. Now I am not talking about someone owning retail stores and having the luxury of making additional income merchandizing and selling fat (Sorry, a futile attempt at humor). I am talking about the sickening, repulsive, addition of fat to one's body.

"So," you say. Well, I think most of us would agree that laziness is part of an individual's personality, part of their character. So one of the reasons people are grotesquely overweight is their personality and the character trait of laziness. Like stated previously, a lazy person does not burn as many calories thus increasing the likelihood of obesity. A comparison would be why does someone not brush his or her teeth on a regular basis? It is the same thing; a person doesn't brush their teeth because they either don't care about their teeth or they are too lazy to brush regularly.

Now how does this justify how we view fat people? Let me ask you this; how do we view people who don't dress nice? People who wear dirty and wrinkled clothing when at their jobs or in situations that call for presentable clothing? No, not cool (I guess I am showing my age here). We view people such as those who don't dress appropriately as being lazy or apathetic with respect to their appearance. Do we view these individuals in a positive light? Do we respect these people for dressing so poorly? No, we don't. And the same lack of respect should be given to individuals who let their body go to hell. Individuals who, due to laziness (or the other causes of obesity), are too lazy to have prevented their obesity should be treated with less respect than someone who takes care of their body. These obese people should have a tag on their back saying, "I am either lazy, lack self-discipline and self control or I am apathetic with respect to my appearance and health." But I guess the tag on the back is not necessary because the fat ass, the monster thighs, or the huge gut are definite give-aways!

Another comparison to someone obese and their laziness would be that of a person who never or rarely showers. How is not showering the same as someone being obese? For one, a person who doesn't shower doesn't care about their health. This same non-showering person also doesn't care about their body or how others perceive, through sight and smell, their body and thus themselves. This is exactly the same as someone who is too lazy to burn some extra calories. It is the same as someone who is apathetic with respect to their body, who lacks self-dignity, consumes too much food, or just sits around all day lying on the couch.

Just one more comparison; think about people who are too lazy to keep their own house or yard clean. You know, the neighbor who never mows their lawn or weeds the yard. The neighbor who has garbage piled up in their back yard, or worse, their front yard. What do you think of these neighbors? How much do you respect these neighbors who are too lazy to get up and mow the lawn? Or how do you perceive the neighbor who is too lazy to clean their yard of garbage and is actually causing a health hazard to themselves and others? Well, this is the same as an individual being lazy with respect to staying fit; to a person being too lazy to get up off their sorry ass, burning some calories, and not eating so much. The sight of the fat person is a visual eyesore just like the garbage in the yard. An individual who is overly fat is endangering their health just like the lazy neighbor and their garbage. So, above all else, the fact that a person is obese shows the entire world that they are lazy, just like the terrible lazy neighbor.

Before I move on to how self-control and discipline contribute to obesity I would like to further touch upon personality. Another perspective of how being an Overly Fat Person relates to personality and character is what some people do to distinguish themselves from the mainstream, or what some people believe are things that convey an individual's "personality." So what are some things that supposedly are indicators of an individuals true personality? A few examples of what many in our society feel are personality indicators are the car a person drives and clothing a person wears; if the person has tattoos and if so what style or where on the body are the tattoos located. And of course there is a person's hairstyle, which most of us feel reveals much in the way of personality. So if people, if many in our society believe these examples just given relate to individuals personality, then how is being fat not a personality indicator? And this is funny! You would think that a fundamentally sound (mentally) individual would believe that the condition of a persons body has more to do with personality then clothing, cars, etc. But not in our fat society, no, the car you drive and the clothes you wear are "you." **What a travesty of intelligent thought!**

Many people say that the car you drive reflects your personality. But the car you drive is not "YOU." Your body is you! The car you drive might indicate your personal preference for cars. The car you drive might indicate how much income you make, although I have seen

15

many people who drive very expensive cars but live in inexpensive run down houses or in small apartments. If you drive a SUV or big truck it somehow indicates (to some people) that you are a tough' macho' guy; yet many petite housewives drive an SUV or trucks. You might think you are flashy and sexy if you drive a sports care. But are you sexy or flashy if you are a fat disgusting pig and drive a sports car? Your body speaks volumes!

Many people try to distinguish themselves with tattoos on their bodies thus offering a form of self-expression to the viewing public. Many people, who in my opinion have an 'Identity Crisis" wear weird clothes or style their hair in a unique fashion. But what is more indicative of who you are then the shape of your body? It identifies that you take pride in yourself. Staying in shape shows that you care about your health. It typically shows that you are not lazy and of course have some semblance of self-control and discipline.

SELF-CONTROL AND DISCIPLINE

WELL, WE HAVE COVERED LAZINESS, NOW lets explore how lacking self-control or discipline with respect to food and drink comes into play with an individual being classified as an "Overly Fat Person." It is sad that I must explain this to readers, as the self-control and obesity relationship should be crystal clear to any sound minded individual. But hey, look at all the fat people rationalizing their disgusting condition.

If one is too believe the "calories in, calories out" theory with respect to obesity (and if you haven't yet figured it out, this is a theory I am behind 100%) then it is blatantly obvious that the self-control and discipline of an individual is a major contributing factor to their obesity. If every time a person sits down to eat they can't control themselves as to the amount of food they ingest then this person will become fat. How overly plain and simple can this be? And my point is that most people consider someone who exhibits self-discipline as a person who has strong character or a strong willed personality. So obviously there is a relationship between obesity and a person's character.

This self-discipline factor comes into play constantly. Not only at the dinner table/ normal meal times but also throughout an individuals waking day. Self-discipline comes into play when the temptation to snack exists/arises. Self-discipline is involved with the overcoming of peer pressure when at a business birthday party and your fellow employees are giving you hell because you pass on the birthday cake. Control and will power come into play at the movies when there is the temptation of the candy and buttered popcorn. Control is necessary when shopping at your local store when they have all the free food samples at the end of the aisles.

As I did with laziness I will now offer some comparisons with respect to individuals who exhibit limited self-control and how we perceive them. A comparison in our society of an "Overly Fat Persons" lack of self-discipline and how we should perceive them would be that of a criminal. Do we respect individuals who steal, commit fraud, murder and rape because of their lack of self–control? Do we respect individuals who lose their temper in the workplace, in public or with the family? Do we respect individuals who break their marriage vows because they don't have the self-control or discipline to avoid the temptation of an affair? (Well maybe, kind of depends on what is, is, doesn't it?) Do we respect individuals who lack the self-control necessary to NOT abuse their spouse or family. The answer to these questions is NO. And the answer to the question of whether we should respect "Overly Fat People" because they lack the self-control and discipline with respect to caloric intake is a resounding NO!

APATHY

AND LASTLY, THE PERSONALITY TRAIT THAT I feel is the most reprehensible with respect to fat people is that of apathy. There are people out there who don't give a damn how obese they become or even how their condition of obesity negatively affects their health. Many of these people hide the fact that they don't care about their bodies or their health through rationalization. And we have heard them all; from, "I am genetically predisposed to obesity," to, "it's a hormone issue" to, "my mom was fat" or that, "I have two kids." These are all copouts and there are millions of examples, both nationally and worldwide, to prove that these rationalizations are indeed just copouts. The bottom line is that if a person doesn't care about and respect "themselves" then why should we? If a person has no dignity towards himself or herself then why in the world should we respect them?

So in conclusion, how should our society perceive, treat, and react to Overly Fat People? How should our society perceive individuals who just don't give a damn about their bodies and are lazy, lack discipline, or are apathetic? The same way we perceive any individual who has these same character issues. We should treat Overly Fat Persons with less respect than a healthy fit person because these obese people have, within their power, the ability to prevent and overcome their condition of obesity.

IF YOU ARE OVERWEIGHT...

YOU ARE NOT:

"LARGE"

YOU ARE NOT:

A "PLUS SIZE"

YOU ARE NOT:

"FLUFFY"

YOU ARE FAT!

CONTROL YOURSELF!!!!!!!!!!!

REMEMBER!!!!!!! IF YOU ARE FAT IT IS BECAUSE OF ONE OR MORE OF THE FOLLOWING:

You are lazy and inactive

You lack any discipline or self-control with respect to food and drink

You are apathetic with respect to your physical condition…. You don't give a damn.

Chapter Three

GENETICS

WELL NOW, THIS CHAPTER ON GENETICS is probably one of the most important chapters in this entire book. Why is this? Genetics is important because of the limited role genetics actually plays in a person being obese. But yet in our society genetics is one of the most often used rationalizations for the condition of obesity. So it is imperative that the genetic rationalization for obesity be dispelled.

It is of significant importance the role of genetics plays with respect to American societies new view of being fat. Americans new view of being obese is that of accepting it as "everybody is different" (genetics) or, "we are not all meant to be thin" (genetics) or it is "entirely genetic" or 'it is natural to become fat as we age" and these views are causing more and more Americans to become very fat. This "genetics" view is allowing millions and millions of Americans to have yet another form of rationalization with respect to their being disgustingly fat due to laziness, lack of self-discipline or apathy.

But I feel that rationalization is actually too nice of a term. Using the word "rationalization" softens the meaning just as "plump" or "Big and Beautiful" softens the meaning of fat or obese. In reality, the genetic rationalization is just an excuse to be totally out of control and do anything you want with respect to food and drink with no regard for the consequences. How often have you heard some fat person state that it, "runs in the family" or, " I guess I was born this way!" But this is just nonsense! An individual is fat because they are totally disrespecting their body and can't control their own over indulgence in food.

Don't believe me? Well let me put forth this scenario. Let's put some fat people in a lifeboat lost at sea for a few months. Everyday all the people must be rowing and occasionally having to bail for their lives during rough seas. The people on the lifeboat are doing this physical activity all the while sustaining themselves on less than 500 calories a day. They continue this hardship and deprivation for at least a couple of weeks, maybe a month or two. **Do you really think that some people on this lifeboat will not lose weight?** REALLY? Give me a break! Everyone on the boat will lose weight. Everyone on the lifeboat will lose a different percentage of his or her body weight and at different rates but everyone will lose weight. So, for an individual to not try to lose weight or for an individual to fail to attempt to maintain a reasonably healthy body because of perceived genetic factors is a cop-out!

Still believe genetics is the major factor in obesity? Well, another example used a few times in this book is this; think about 1941 or 1942 Stalingrad and tell me if you think there were a lot of fat people amongst the German or Russian Armies or within the civilian population (view old films and photos)? Why is that? Do you honestly believe that all these people in and around Stalingrad in 1942 were thin due to genetics? Do you think these soldiers and civilians were genetically **predisposed to thinness?** Yeah, right! They were thin and emancipated due to lack of food! Get the picture? "Calories in, calories out." Ever hear of that???????

Another thing I hear quite often with respect to the importance of genetics in obesity is a comparison of families. This family is all thin; this family is all fat, it must be related to genetics! This automatically attributing the obesity in the one family to genetics is absurd! Why on earth do people automatically suspect genetics as the culprit? Does it not occur to anyone that the entire family is fat due to their living and eating habits? Think not? Well, take one member of an obese family and put them in our previously mentioned lifeboat scenario. Do you think the fat family member would lose weight or would this fat person body stay basically the same? This fat family member would indeed lose weight and this is yet another example of what limited role genetics plays in an individual or families condition of obesity.

Now, I can just hear some of you critics out there saying I am incorrect, especially after reading further in the book other chapters such as the chapter on Competitiveness or the chapter on Sports. You will feel that I am contradicting myself. How, on one hand can I emphasize the importance of genetics dealing with the likelihood of an individual becoming a world-class athlete, and on the other hand minimize the impact of genetics with respect to obesity? My answer is this, "I don't care what you think".... JUST KIDDING! So lets examine the "If a person has little control over having the capability to be a world-class athlete, then a person has little control over whether they will become fat." Well, to a certain degree they are correct. You can't make an Alberto Salazar (former world class distance runner) into a Bo Jackson or Hershel Walker (two extremely athletic and well muscled Former NFL running backs). But we can all be or have some semblance of physical fitness and muscle tone. Some of us are genetically inclined to be like the distance runner. Some of us are genetically inclined to be like the Pro Football player. And most of us are genetically inclined to be somewhere in-between the distance runner and the pro football player. But, although some of us may not be able to reduce our fat content below certain percentage levels we can all avoid obesity. We all have the capability to avoid obesity! We all have the capability to avoid becoming an OFP. And the examples in the previous paragraphs prove my point. Just hop on that lifeboat if you don't believe me!

Genetics also comes into play in another manner. Many people use the genetics excuse in a "feel sorry for myself" way. An "OFP" may state, "Sally can eat all she wants and doesn't get fat, so I will eat as much as her and if I become fat it is natural for me, it is my genetics." For a person to rationalize their fatness because they can't lose weight as easily as others is a "cop-out." It's like a person letting themselves get fat because their best friend can eat 5000 calories a day and not gain a pound and they themselves can only eat about 2000 calories a day without gaining weight. That is the same rationale as being in a high school math class and sitting next to the whiz kid who doesn't have/need to study but still gets A's. Should you not study like the whiz kid and fail your math class? Or should you realize that life is not always fair and buckle down and study? Of course you should study! And of course you should limit your caloric intake to maintain some form of physical dignity. You should only eat what you can eat without getting fat! If you do indeed eat more then what your body needs it is because of your personality and the fact that you are either lazy, have no self control with respect to food or that you just don't have the dignity and self-respect to care about your body.

In conclusion, genetics plays a very, very limited role in our nations obesity epidemic. For individuals to rely on the genetics rationalization as an excuse for their reprehensible condition is despicable.

IF YOU'RE A FAT AND DISGUSTING IT'S YOUR FAULT!

CHANGE!

IF YOU ARE OVERWEIGHT

YOU ARE NOT:

"VOLUMPTOUS"

YOU ARE NOT:

"BIG BONED"

ALLTHOUGH YOU CAN BE BIG BONED AND NOT FAT!

YOU ARE NOT:

"CURVEY"

YOU ARE FAT!

REMEMBER!!!!!! IF YOU ARE FAT IT IS BECAUSE OF ONE OR MORE OF THE FOLLOWING:

You are lazy and inactive.

You lack any discipline or self-control with respect to food and drink.

You are apathetic with respect to your physical condition…. You don't give a damn.

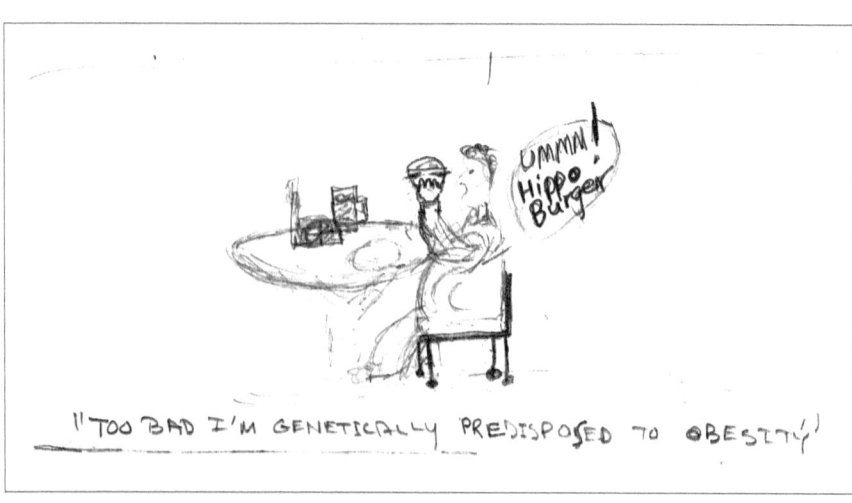

"TOO BAD I'M GENETICALLY PREDISPOSED TO OBESITY"

Chapter Four

SOCIETAL INFLUENCES

OUR SOCIETY HAS MUCH TO BLAME with respect to our nations obesity epidemic. The first influence I will relate to is how we perceive an individuals body and whether or not this individual is fat.

VISUAL PERCEPTION

OUR PERCEPTION OF WHAT IS "FAT" is much different now than when I was a child or even a young adult. For instance, in the 1970's I would often enjoy watching the *Mary Tyler Moore* show. I remember Lou Grant looking extremely fat and overweight. As I watch reruns/discs of the show now, Lou doesn't appear as fat as before. Hmmm. Have they doctored the disc? Did Lou and everybody get back together and re-film the show? How about Mary, how did she appear? When I recently watched the show, I believe it was the first or second season, I thought to myself, "wow, Mary is skinny." But back in the 1970's I don't remember ever thinking that Mary was skinny or too slender.

Do you remember *Bonanza*? How did Hoss look back in those days? Do you remember him? Now I don't know what your perception was back then but myself, along with all my classmates and friends, thought Hoss was fat. Hoss may have been strong as an ox but yet he still was fat. Now, when I watch a *Bonanza* episode, Hoss doesn't strike me as being so overweight, at least not to the degree perceived years ago. But then again, you, along with me, are becoming accustomed and conditioned to looking at fat people.

We are becoming conditioned to being fat, looking fat, looking at others who are fat and perceiving this as "NORMAL." It is similar to how we feel now when we look at someone with a shaved head or see someone wearing shorts down to or below their knees. (Shorts will reach the ankles soon, I'm sure.) We are accustomed to it…. It is normal. But what would we have thought back in the 1970's if someone had worn shorts that went down below the knee or lower? What did we think of people who were bald or shaved their heads? What did we think and how did we perceive Telly Savalas in *Kojak*? What did we think of the actor Yul Brynner? How about the basketball player Slick Watts?

If you don't think we, as Americans are fat and just becoming accustomed to seeing fat individuals, just do some traveling overseas. When you return I bet one of the things you will notice is that there are great numbers of Americans who are fat. And unfortunately/conversely, if you are fat and you travel overseas you just might think that everyone over there is skinny and that you are normal. This is one of our nations biggest problems; being fat is becoming normal and is accepted amongst our society.

ADVERTISING

ANOTHER SOCIETAL INFLUENCING FACTOR WITH RESPECT to obesity is that of today's advertising. Advertising is indeed an area of concern with respect to our nation becoming a haven for "Overly Fat

People." Take television advertising for example. Do you realize how inundated we are with commercials that advertise something that contains calories? Be it commercials for restaurants, both fast food and fine dinning, to beer or other alcohol commercials, we are bombarded with images and messages to eat and drink. Even commercials that are not advertising food often have images of people eating and drinking, preparing food in the kitchen or barbecuing. Our society is overwhelmed by food, food, and food, eat, eat, and eat. With this constant bombardment of food related advertising is it surprising that so many individuals eat too much? Is it surprising that people trying to lose weight have difficulty because their mind is always thinking about food?

Another problem with advertising (and also of television and films) and how it is contributing to the fat culture is that of using fat actors and actresses for more movies and commercials than in previous years. Why is this happening? I am not sure! (well, there is the "fat market" demographic that must be appealing to advertisers) What problem does this pose? To that, I am sure! This using of fat people in advertising and on television in general is further reinforcing the view that it is natural to be overweight. It expresses the notion that some fat 250-pound woman is beautiful and that all women have permission to just let their bodies go to hell. That all people should just eat however much they want and that they are still beautiful. Stuff your face to your hearts content!!!!!!!!

FOOD PORTIONS

ANOTHER FACTOR IN OUR SOCIETY THAT contributes to obesity is the amount/size of food portions. Food portions have dramatically increased over the years and this increase of calories at every meal is making us fat. Do any of you remember how big a hamburger was at McDonalds back in the 1960's? Much smaller then a Big Mac now, I guarantee you. How about the size of a typical soft drink?

Of course we as individuals could use self-discipline and purchase smaller meals or save some of the large meal for later, but no!

The sad part is, back in the 60's restaurants didn't have to serve large portions because the average person couldn't finish a meal as large as today's typical meal. I bet those of you who lived in the 60's or 70's back then would have had extreme difficulty downing a foot long sub sandwich. How many of us can say that now? Most adult males in our society have no difficulty at all in finishing off a foot long sandwich in one sitting. Our whole society; our whole culture, is becoming accustomed to devouring extremely large portions of food at one sitting.

And of course what does all this mean? It means if you lack self-discipline around food or are just apathetic about your body and health you will finish the large serving that is presented to you and thus intake much, much more in the way of calories then you should to remain fit and healthy.

FOOD ASSOCIATIONS

Not only are food portions greater now and are causing problems in relation to obesity but also food is everywhere and associated with everything. What can an American do without having to consume food? If you and your family sit down and watch television what do you have to have to enjoy yourselves? You have to have something to snack on or literally "pig out" on. Think of what is common to eat when watching football games with your friends. Not that we should have to eat something to enjoy a football game but a couple of large pizzas is not uncommon. Also common would be multiple bags of chips, some beer (probably a lot of beer) and maybe some pizza.

What if you go to a sporting event? Yes, you must have your food fix. Even if it means spending ten times the amount of money for food and drink as elsewhere, you have to have the food. I mean, how can you enjoy a baseball game without a beer and hotdog, right? How about a movie? You must have that buttered popcorn in the container that should feed four. Of course, it's just the two of you; and of course, even if you get full you must finish the popcorn as otherwise it would be a waste of money.

Of course it's different if you are participating in a sport, right? WRONG! How about you golfers? Gotta bring along or purchase the booze to drink on the course. You also must have that energy bar or candy bar to help you survive those 4 hours without food. And then there is the 19th green; that's where you can replenish your food stores before going home to dinner in a few hours.

What about you softball players? Do you belong to a league where beer and other foods are prevalent? What about some, and I mean some, of you bike riders? How much do you pack along for a two-hour bike ride? (I know... I am well aware most avid cyclists are in great shape...)

Where and when else do we have to have food when it is not necessary? How about those little road trips you take. How many of you can drive for more than two hours without having to stop for some food or break out the reserves? Give me a break! If we as humans can't even go without food or drink for two hours then we have a problem. And yes, we do have a problem.

How many of us can even go shopping without eating something? How about when you go to a store such as Costco? Think of those demonstrators handing out the samples of food? How many of us can resist the temptation to try the samples? Not just the samples where we really don't have any idea of how the food tastes, but all of the samples. You would think we are starving as a nation when you observe the people lining up for the free samples. Food, food, food! It's pathetic, but it is a direct microcosm of how the average American reacts to food. I believe if there was free food and we could tie food around people's necks in a feedbag then people would just keep eating. It is pathetic, disgusting and revolting.

But all of these before mentioned examples are part of our accepted society. And all of these examples help explain why so many in our nation are, or will become, fat and obese.

RIDICULE-PEER PRESURE

How ELSE CAN OUR SOCIETY AFFECT our body weight and lead individuals down the path of destruction, thus becoming an OFP? How about when you are with friends and co-workers? Think not; well how about at the office meeting or party? What happens when you politely refuse to eat some cake or other food? Well, if you're a man I can tell you what because I have experienced it myself. You will get the comments like, "Oh, you are watching your girlish figure." Or you will hear, "Come on, you're not fat." Well, compared to the people who just criticized you, you are probably not fat. But it never occurs to these Overly Fat People that the reason you are **not** fat is because you have some self-restraint. That one of the reasons you are not fat is because when someone offers you some food, you don't automatically accept. That, yes indeed, you are watching your weight and you are indeed proud of being in good shape.

The funny thing is that it is all right for these fat souls to criticize you for not eating and trying to either maintain your weight or reduce your weight but heaven forbid if you were to say something to a fat person with respect to eating that same birthday cake. That same fat person would probably report you to the Human Resource Department for abusive and/or discriminatory behavior if you, as a normal person, were to say something like, " are you sure you need that second piece of cake?" This is sadly true because now it is more politically correct and normal in our society to be fat and critical of people who are thin or even just normal and want to stay that way then it is for someone, heaven forbid, to tell a fat person that maybe they should just resist that piece of birthday cake. How very sad!

For males there is also the pressure from society to "eat like a man." If a man doesn't want to down some bratwurst or a big fat juicy hamburger when watching the game with his buddies he will be ridiculed. If a man lets on to other supposedly macho guys that he likes Sushi or Sashimi then he will be teased. More on this subject latter in the chapter" I am A Man."

WORDS

LET'S ALSO EXAMINE SOCIETIES RE-TAKE ON words and phrases. This is done all the time in our country to help alleviate any stigma surrounding a group of people. This changing of vocabulary usage has been done with respect to retarded people, in education, with respect to minority groups, etc.

First, some examples of words of which the meanings have changed but that are not fat related. These examples may also add some levity. I am sure after the Civil War that it was not meant that we will all be Homosexuals (Gay) " When Johnny Comes Marching Home." And I am sure that the term "Booty" had a different connotation to pirates back in the day then it has now.

Now lets think about what words we presently use to describe fat people. One of the words/terms that bothers me the most is the term "Full Figured." For anyone over 40 years of age it is quite apparent that this term has changed tremendously over the years. "Full Figured" previously meant or related to women who were significantly endowed with respect to their breasts. Names that come to mind of women who fell into this category are Jane Russell, Raquel Welch and other large breasted but thin/normal women. The key is thin (by today's standards because back then thin was normal) and large breasted. Unfortunately today "Full Figured" is some fat culture rationalization and de-stigmatizing term for women who can't control themselves around food and drink. "We can't control ourselves and have fat bodies, but we need to somehow gain respect from others who are not as disgustingly over indulgent as ourselves, "state the fat women." Fat women state, we can't think of ourselves as fat, which would be depressing, so we think of ourselves as "Full Figured." Yeah, great for our country, huh! (See the end of chapters for examples of other "words" that attempt to de-stigmatize)

So all this softening of words that minimize the impact of obesity is another way society is contributing to the fat epidemic that is destroying our country.

SPORTS

SPORTS HAVE DEFINITELY INFLUENCED HOW THE modern day American views him or herself and what is appropriate with respect to body type and behavior. The increased popularity of pro wrestling, mixed martial arts and football lead us to believe that what we are seeing is the ideal body type. This might be true! It might be entirely true that we all want to look like Terrell Owens or some huge and ripped martial artist. The problem lies in when we as individuals hear the **height and weights** of these individuals and forget that a great percentage of these athletes weight is muscle! Another problem is that most of these individuals are either genetic abnormalities (desirable in a culturally perceived way) or are ingesting something into their bodies to enhance their shape and muscularity. But like, "being a man" "sports" also has a chapter in this book; so more on sports and its influence on society later.

HUSBAND AND WIFE

WELL, HOW MANY TIMES HAVE WE heard it, especially from guys, "I was thin till I got married, my wife just cooks too good." There is a lot of truth to that statement and often times the statement is made as a statement of fact as opposed to an excuse or rationalization. But for whatever reason the statement is made and for what ever the cause the fact remains when people get married many of them get fat.

One cause for this fact of many people becoming fat because of marriage probably lies in the old, "well, I am married now, it doesn't matter if my body goes to hell, I don't have to attract a mate... so what if I don't look as good?"

This next reason for marriage contributing to obesity that I am about to mention can occur in an old-fashioned traditional type marriage or even in less tradition/non-conforming situations. But I believe an even larger cause for weight gain after being married is that both spouses love each other. Yes, because they love each other they contribute to each other's obesity. One spouse wants nothing more then to make the other spouse happy. So one spouse might always cook great meals for the other spouse; meals that are extravagant and probably too large portion wise, just to make their spouse pleased, happy or content. And of course the spouse not doing the cooking feels obligated to consume everything placed in front of them as to show appreciation and love. So what is meant as a gestures of love, actually could be contributing to one or both spouse's demise (think about that at the dinner table after just naming your spouse as beneficiary on a life insurance policy). And actually, when one spouse is eating a lot food the other spouse is probably following right along. What a great situation!

The remedy to this husband and wife contributing to each other's obesity is quite simple. So, like the basic requirements for staying normal, all the husband and wife need is some discipline. It might also be necessary for the cook of the family to realize there is more then one way to a person's heart and that large portions of food is not the answer. Food is not the best way to a person's heart if you indeed truly love that person. If you truly love your spouse you care about their health and well-being and causing your spouse to become obese is a cruel way to show your love!

In conclusion, there are many things in our society that contribute to our nations fat epidemic. Many factors exist and I am sure that I probably missed many factors that are obvious to you the reader. But the important thing is to be aware that society is influencing individuals in our society and that we, as a nation, ought to find ways to remedy this sad situation.

IF YOU ARE OVERWEIGHT

YOU ARE NOT:

"HEAVY"

YOU ARE NOT:

"FULL FIGURED"

Full figure used to mean the figures of women such as Jane Russell or Raquel Welch, not fat women!

YOU ARE NOT:

"HEFTY"

YOU ARE FAT!

YOU ARE A FAT SLOB!

REMEMBER!!!!!!! IF YOU ARE FAT IT IS BECAUSE OF ONE OR MORE OF THE FOLLOWING:

You are lazy and inactive.

You lack any discipline or self-control with respect to food and drink.

You are apathetic with respect to your physical condition…. You don't give a damn.

Chapter Five

PREGNANCY

BOY, DON'T WOMEN JUST LOVE TO use anything that is exclusive to women as an excuse for everything. And heaven help any male who questions these excuses. And boy, don't I just love alienating large segments of our society? Among women "pregnancy" and "hormone" rationalizations with respect to being fat is somewhat prevalent. And often times the hormone rationalization to why one is fat is also tied to previous pregnancy or pregnancies or to postpartum depression. You hear this pregnancy rationalization all the time from fat women. But sorry women, this is a sad excuse for your obesity.

HORMONES

I KNOW, I KNOW. WHAT DO I know, I am a man? Well, should this fact not allow me to make rational and objective observations with respect to women? Should women not be allowed to make any observations of men strictly because they aren't men and don't have the large amounts of testosterone streaming through their veins like that in men?

It's funny because women always use the hormone excuse. Well, us guys should start doing this also. Hey, let women try to deal with our high levels of testosterone. For instance, does a woman know what it's like when I am walking down the sidewalk of downtown Portland on a hot summers day with a breeze blowing and I am following two slim teenage girls wearing mini-skirts? Do they realize the self-control that a warm blooded American male must exhibit when facing these hormonal scenarios?

But of course guys can't use their hormones as an excuse. "Excuse me babe, I was just walking behind you and the breeze blew and your skirt kind of raised up and your behind looked so nice I just had to "cop a feel." "It's my hormones you know." Yea, right. A guy would get sent to jail for that touch, unless of course it was a very understanding young woman.

So the point is that women should not use hormones and even pregnancy as an excuse to become a grotesquely obese human. Want more reasons and observations why pregnancy should not be an excuse for obesity? Of course you do!

Well now, go take a vacation to Japan. Take a look at the women there. I have taken at least 5 trips to Japan and have spent many a day observing the physical features of the Japanese women (this was *hard* work). And guy's, if you like slender (by American standards) women, Japan is a great place to go, but back to the point. Not only are there many normal or slender, by American standards, single women in Japan but there are many, many women *with children* who are not obese. Millions!

Another observation that should be made and an observation that is very noteworthy is taking a look at athletes who have been pregnant. If I had ever thought I would be writing a book such as this I would have taken notes… But for most of my life, until maybe the last ten years, I actively followed track and field. And there were many women runners who stopped their training to have a child and then returned to compete. And, in a very short period of time, compete quite well I might add. And if you have ever watched World Class runners (I will omit from this the female shot-putters and discus throwers) they are never even close to being overweight.

So why is this? How come Japanese women can have numerous kids and not get fat? How come runners can have kids and not get fat? What is their secret? Don't you dare say "genetics!"

Well, as is the case in most weight loss scenarios, there is no secret. It is "calories in- calories out." With respect to the Japanese women and the runners remaining thin/normal after pregnancy there is that one thing they have to their advantage and that is they were probably not fat when they became pregnant. Can all you American women who are using your pregnancy as an excuse for your obesity claim the same? Can you fat American women who are now fat after pregnancy claim that you were thin/normal before something starting baking in the oven? Well, I bet a large percentage cannot. And you women who had shapely figures before pregnancy should think about all the runners, other female athletes and Japanese women who quickly regain their figures after their pregnancy.

EATING FOR TWO

Now PREVIOUSLY, I HAD BEEN HARPING on the hormone factor. And obviously this hormone factor comes into play during pregnancy. So what do a lot of women do when they're pregnant? They binge on various delicacies and use either the hormone excuse or they state, " I am eating for two."

Well, in the first instance, relating to the hormones, women just need to use a little self-control. Get a life!!!!! Are women, and men also, just animals and should give in to any and all urges whether or not from hormones? Of course we should not. So women, get a handle on it, all right. How about just using some self-control.

With respect to the eating for two, a common rationalization for pregnant women, well that is a joke! That is a rationalization that causes many women to get fat or even fatter while pregnant. And this is not just the author's opinions, observations or theories. It is now basically common knowledge by most of the medical community that a women only needs a few hundred extra calories (AT MOST) a day for her fetus to be healthy. Some experts state that, especially in the early stages of pregnancy that NO ADDITIONAL calories are needed, just good nutrition. Just two or three hundred extra calories (that's just three light beers or two martinis! Just kidding…). Do you realize how little, with respect to quantity of food, two or three hundred extra calories is? How many women who have become fat during pregnancy consume much, much more than 200 to 300 extra calories? Many, if not all! So guess why these women get fat?

One other factor comes into play for women who are pregnant. And that is activity level. Unless there are unusual circumstances and or complications there is no reason a woman can't remain physically active through almost her entire pregnancy. There have been women who have run marathons when 6 months or more pregnant. But of course, in our lazy and rationalistic prone society, being pregnant is just another excuse for sitting on your ass and eating too much.

Get a life!

POSTPARTUM DEPRESSION

WELL, I WAS AT WORK THE other day and one of my co-workers started going off on postpartum depression and how terrible it is for women. First, I would like to state that I am not denying the existence of postpartum depression; all I want to state is that it should not be used as an excuse for women becoming obese after pregnancy. How can a "man" say this! What does a man know?

My stance on postpartum depression is the same as women battling hormones when pregnant. I guess the millions of women in Japan, who are slender by American standards, and maintained that slenderness/normalcy after bearing children must be immune from this terrible condition of postpartum depression that causes American women to become fat! And I guess all the women pro athletes who kept their shape during (except the belly of course) and after pregnancy never had to overcome postpartum depression, huh?

In short, I am not minimizing the condition of Postpartum depression, I am only stating that if millions of women around the world and in the U.S. can have a normal shape after pregnancy then so can others! Use some self-control and stop rationalizing.

HEALTH

OF ANOTHER MAJOR CONCERN OF SOMEONE either being obese before pregnancy or of becoming obese during pregnancy due to rationalization or lack of self-control around food and drink is the issue of health. It is unhealthy for both the mother and the child if the mother is obese when pregnant. I cover more of the ramifications of obesity while pregnant in the chapter on health.

IF YOU ARE OVERWEIGHT…

YOU ARE NOT:

"HEAVY"

YOU ARE NOT:

"FULL FIGURED"

YOU ARE NOT:

"CHUBBY"

YOU ARE FAT!

GET A LIFE!

REMEMBER!!!!!!! IF YOU ARE FAT IT IS BECAUSE OF ONE OR MORE OF THE FOLLOWING:

You are lazy and inactive.

You lack any discipline or self-control with respect to food and drink.

You are apathetic with respect to your physical condition…. You don't give a damn.

Chapter Six

I 'M A MAN!

WELL, WITH A CHAPTER ON PREGNANCY, which is obviously devoted to women (I believe even Gay Rights activists will agree to this fact), I thought I would add some interesting perspectives to problems men face and how it is common for men to rationalize their obesity with the "I am a man" rationale.

Much of this chapter could be, and some is, included in the Society chapter and the chapter on Sports. But, like I just mentioned, if I ripped on the women, well then I better hurry-up and rip on the men. So how does a male's perceived image of a "man," or better yet, an American man, relate to obesity?

Now, I am about to generalize here, and I am aware that this is very dangerous. Dangerous indeed! But being an American male and having American male friends (at least before the publication of this book) I am aware of how a good portion of the American public perceives the ideal American male with respect to body type. Yes, I am aware that all the thin distance runners, thin tennis players and other males who think lifting a weight is some perverse activity might think differently; but most men think that if they could, that they would like to be like the average pro football or pro basketball player. I am referring to a male about 6'2" to 6'5", weighing (although weight is not important but strength and definition are) about 200 to 240 pounds with measurables of 20 plus repetitions of the combine weight (225lbs. for you non-football types) 4.5 speed or better in a 40 and a vertical leap of 40 plus inches.

What is wrong with this you ask? **Absolutely nothing!!!!!!!!!!!!!!!!!!!!** And if every American male strived to achieve such standards and attempted to look chiseled and like a rock, then there would be no problem. Our Society would be a much better place both from a visual perspective and from a health perspective. But from the previous example of the ideal athlete many American males seem to forget the strength and definition aspect of standing 6'2" and weighing 200 or so pounds! Through selective listening, a fat man only hears the weight of the pro football player, and forgets that most of that football players weight is in muscle. This is just one of the problems.

Additionally, what has happened to the perceived image of an American male is that it has become perceived as more "manly" and "tough" to be heavy as opposed to thin. The average male in America who weighs over 200 pounds and is fat, not well conditioned, actually feels he is more of "a man" then lets say a 160-pound male who is into distance running or tennis or whatever. There are many reasons for this and most are totally insane.

One of the reasons a 200 pound out of shape or obese male thinks he is more manly than the man of slighter build is that of perceived toughness or fighting ability. But take it from someone who has had 3 years of martial arts training and has personally witnessed some incredible feats of athleticism and fighting prowess, that physical size is only important if all other variables are equal. This importance of size has more to do with height and reach and muscular weight as opposed to fat weight. The other variables I mentioned are fighting ability and training and natural gifts such as reflexes, strength, coordination and fighting strategy. Of course, don't mention these facts to a fat slob that thinks he is tough. And I should mention, that yes indeed, a person can be a fat slob and be "tough" and a good fighter! But this same person could be tough and a good fighter without all the excess weight. So lose the fat, man!

Don't believe me? How would you, Mr. 225 pound ball of blubber with limited training with respect to fighting, like to fight the ghost of Bruce Lee? How would you manly but somewhat pudgy guy like to fight any of the world class Welterweight or Middleweight fighters of today? How about fighting just some everyday 160 pound guy who has black belts in a couple of different martial art disciplines?

So my point is simply that just because you are bigger/heavier then the next guy, in most likely hood (statistically speaking in our entire male population), it does not mean you are more of a man, a better or tougher fighter, or anything else for that matter.

Returning to the Pro Football player example, most Pro Football players are in great shape. As mentioned previously in this book there is 6'2" and 230 pounds and there is 6'2" and 230 pounds. This is the other part of the problem. A guy listening to a Pro Football game on television hears the announcers give heights and weights all the time. The listener becomes conditioned to hearing these heights and weights (see chapter on sports) and forgets that probably 90% of these football players are built like a tank, like a rock. But all the listener hears is the height and weight! So when Mr. Obesity steps on the scales and sees his weight his thought is not, "Boy, I need to lose some pounds," but his thought is more along the lines of, " well that's not so bad, just like an average NFL linebacker." Yeah, right!!!!!!!!!!!! Of course this obese individual conveniently avoids gazing in the mirror when naked or without a shirt! That would be too life like and might necessitate some re-evaluation with respect to himself; that might require some self-discipline, that might require getting up off their fat you know what (no, I am not afraid to use the word Ass) and actually doing something.

Let's take another issue of a heavy overweight (not well built but overweight) guy feeling he is more of a man than lets say a 150 pound tone runner. Hey, Mr. Obese, do you think performance in bed is any indicator of manhood? Gee, even if your gay, performance in bed must be an indicator of something, right? (This last remark made not knowing if Gay's like to think of themselves as "Macho") But who do you think will perform better in bed (not considering technique or physical endowments, personality, facial features that arouse their partner, etc.) an obese male or a thin male? As far as being able to physically last longer I think the answer is obvious. But don't forget the reaction of the female (and to appease all diverse groups, the reaction of the male, dog, inflatable doll, etc.). Gee, would the average woman rather have a fat, extremely obese man on top or be looking down at some fat guys blubber (yes I know, there is also from behind) bouncing or would she rather be in bed with a male that is fit? Well, what's your answer, you "OFP" of the male gender?

There is also another problem for the "Man." This is the problem that it is perceived "manly" to down a lot of food, and even worse yet, eat a lot of food that is high in calories (Fat is also unhealthy but I am primarily concerned with weight…"calories in, calories out"). For example, it is considered manly to, when at a tailgate party or a barbecue or whatever, stuff one's face full of all sorts of high calorie foods. And even worse, heaven help a man who refuses an additional hotdog, brat, hamburger, steak etc., for he will be considered by many less of a "real man."

Heaven help a guy who at a business party or meeting refuses some cake or other high calorie food. A standard reply will be, " what's wrong, you watching your girly figure?" Watching your girly figure, is that not a hit on a male's masculinity?

For a male there is even the problem of eating light at restaurants or at the previously mentioned business functions. It is perfectly fine for a woman to eat the salad or say she is on a diet. But if a man states he is on a diet there are usually the smirks, the chuckles and the thinking this guy must be weird or something.

In short, it is tough being a guy… much tougher than being a woman. LOL!

IF YOU ARE OVERWEIGHT

YOU ARE NOT:

"PORTLY"

YOU ARE NOT:

"BIG AND BEAUTIFUL"

YOU ARE NOT:

"PLUMP"

YOU ARE FAT!

USE SELF-CONTROL!

REMEMBER !!!!!!! IF YOU ARE FAT IT IS BECAUSE OF ONE OR MORE OF THE FOLLOWING:

You are lazy and inactive

You lack any discipline or self-control with respect to food and drink

You are apathetic with respect to your physical condition…. You don't give a damn.

Chapter Seven

SPORTS

WELL NOW, I SUPPOSE YOU'RE WONDERING what do sports have to contribute to an obesity discussion besides the fact that if you participate in sports on a regular basis you are burning a substantial amount of calories and thus have a better chance of not being an Overly Fat Person? Sports have a definite impact on obesity in our American culture due to how we perceive the human body (read previous chapter). More specifically, since much of the population idolizes the professional athlete, the athlete's body is perceived as a measuring standard for the general population. Sports also have ramifications in our nations obesity epidemic because by studying various sports we can easily determine what sports and activities are most beneficial for reducing an individual's weight. Additionally, sports (I am including various exercises as types of sports) contribute in that they help individuals burn calories and simultaneously keep individuals preoccupied and away from food.

PROFESSIONAL SPORTS IN AMERICA

LETS FIRST LOOK INTO HOW PRO sports influence our society with respect to "ideal" body types. Thus, the question we need to ask ourselves, do professional athletes have bodies that we should idolize? We also should ask ourselves, if indeed we do idolize the bodies of professional athletes, which sports offer the healthiest example and which sports have athletes who have bodies that are genetically obtainable for the average individual?

There exists, in today's society, the problems of respecting or idolizing someone who is excelling at a sport, such as football, and conclude that his or her height and weight are the standard by which we should live. If Mr. Defensive lineman who is 6'5" and weighs 340 pounds is a great football player than why should it not be a great standard for Mr. Joe Blow? And this scenario plays itself out quite often amongst the male population. When it is stated on the air that the Defensive Back is "only" 185 pounds and it is then implied that this is "puny" by the announcers this has repercussions in the male population. The insinuation made by the announces, that if you are only 185 pounds that you are puny and need to gain some weight harms our society. Second, if you are a fat man weighing 200lbs. then you might think of yourself as "fit" or "macho" just from what you have heard from some announcer. And more then likely this announcer is overweight and relishing in the fact that it makes him feel more comfortable with his weight calling someone 185 or 190 pounds skinny or puny.

How many American males think that just because their height and weight match those of some NFL Linebacker that their weight must be reasonable for a man (Sorry, redundancy from the previous chapter, but some casual readers or females may have skipped the "I'm a Man" chapter)? Set aside the fact that the NFL Linebacker they are comparing themselves with is cut out of stone, can bench 30-40 repetitions of the combine weight and also runs a 4.5 or so 40 and can run this speed for extended plays/periods of time. And of course this layman, who is comparing himself to the NFL Linebacker, is a fat slob with a 40-inch waist who would have trouble benching a few reps of their body weight and becomes winded running to the bathroom or refrigerator, let alone play most of a football game.

These are important questions and the answers are many. First, there is 6'5" and 340 and there is 6'5" and 340, meaning you can be a "Rock" at this height and weight and you could also be a fat slob/OFP or you could fall somewhere in-between. Second, even if the professional football player may be a little on the heavy side there can be reasons why the pro keeps his body at this weight. For any of you who have lifted a lot of weights you know that one of the quickest ways to gain strength, but not necessarily a great physique, is to stuff your face with food and supplements and lift weights like a madman. So this facet, the need for strength in a football player may be the reason for their body weight.

I feel an excellent example of the need for more body weight was the last year or so of Warren Sapp's career with the Oakland Raiders. One season with the Raiders Sapp led the league in sacks for interior linemen. That season in which he was on top of his game he probably weighed close to 350 pounds. The next season Sapp played at about 300 pounds after deciding in the off-season to become lighter and healthier. And you guessed it; the season he played at around 300 pounds he was much, much less a force on the football field.

Also, with respect to increased body weight and the football player, there is the factor of feeling more "cushioned" so to speak against blows to the body. So these factors need to be taken into consideration by the layman when he or she is thinking of comparing to him or herself with Mr. Lineman. "I weigh the same as him so I must be o.k. with respect to body fat." Sure!

There is also something I need to say with respect to professional football and its players. I would say roughly 90% of them have bodies I would die for. Most of professional football players are in tremendous physical condition, especially the "skill" players. The only players who sometimes are too heavy are the offensive and defensive linemen. And I want to heavily (no pun intended) emphasize "sometimes" as there are many, many lineman in the NFL who are rock solid. There even have been NFL linemen who have, during the off-season, in their playing days run marathons (I believe it was either Alan Page or Jim Marshal, formerly of the Vikings and Greg Wisniewski, formerly of the Raiders as two examples of lineman having completed marathons). And even if these pro football players are not rock solid the contributing factors previously mentioned coupled with these players ability to earn incomes far beyond the average individual makes their playing weight absurd as far as a comparison for weight standards for the average individual.

SPORTS FOR WEIGHT LOSS ANALYSIS

BUT LET'S LOOK AT ANOTHER REASON the study of sports is relevant to obesity. Sports analysis is important with respect to what the best ways to keep from getting fat and what are the best ways of taking the fat off. Just think about it; it is rather obvious, but who has overall the better body type, a professional soccer player or a professional golfer? I know, I know, look at Tiger Woods. But I am talking about "on average" and I must say, if you don't think Tiger Woods does something besides walking the golf course to stay in shape then you are a fool.

So how does this sports comparison relate to Joe or Sally Blow? Well, what is a better way to stay in shape or to lose weight, walking or running? Guys, take a look at the average women pro soccer player over the age of 25 years of age and take a look at the 25 years of age or older LPGA player and tell me, on average, who would you rather date (or did I mean mate)? I am putting monetary motives aside and I feel that the average guy would rather have the hot date with a female soccer player. Gals, who would you rather spend time with in a hot tub, some possibly flabby golf pro or some pro soccer player who is "cut" and can go forever? Hmmmm.

What should all of this be telling us? It is telling us that running is much better than walking with weight loss in mind. That walking is a great transitional activity; hopefully leading to more vigorous endeavors, but walking does not burn the fat/calories like a good running workout.

Another visual with respect to the world of sports that is helpful in terms of determining the best way to lose weight or to keep weight off is that of the use of a stationary bike. Now I know, you can vary the resistance tremendously on a stationary bike and thus increasing the intensity of the workout. But think of how many times you see a pro athlete using a stationary bike to keep "loose" or keep "warm"? The key word here is "LOOSE." Yes, riding the stationary bike keeps you loose and the blood flowing but it does little more unless you really, really crank up the resistance. What does this tell us? Well, do you see these athletes jogging around the football field (I know this would not be practical or even possible but if it were possible would they?)? No, they wouldn't because it would tire them out too much due to jogging or running being more intense. Thus, running or jogging is much better than riding a stationary bike with respect to burning calories. These observations should be kept in mind for anyone trying to lose or maintain body weight.

SPORTS AND EXERCISE

THE FINAL ASPECT OF SPORTS WITH which I would like to comment relates to sports and exercise and how these activities can aid in controlling obesity. As I have mentioned in other chapters of this book, I believe it is easier to avoid the intake of excessive calories than it is to burn off excessive calories. However, I am also a firm believer that individuals feel much better, are healthier, and maintain a better physical appearance when they exercise. Some information with respect to sports and how sports aid in the fight against obesity is also mentioned in the chapter on Diets And Other Solutions.

The most important concept I would like to mention with relation to sports and losing weight is that the more strenuous the sport the better that sport is for the burning of calories. **This should seem quite obvious**, however, a good portion of our society falls prey to advertising and other information which can lead a person to believe that it's possible to lose massive amounts of weight with some form of light exercise just a few times a week. True, coupled with a good diet with much less caloric intake than normal, light exercise will help a person lose much weight, but the important component of this formula is the **diet,** not the light exercise. If you don't believe me, think back to the examples I have already given such as comparing pro golfers over the age of 25 to that of pro soccer players over the age of 25…who is thinner? Well, the soccer players are thinner even though golfers do a lot of walking and standing. Why is this? It is like I just mentioned, the more strenuous the activity the more calories are burned.

The important concepts to remember in this chapter are that there are few short cuts to losing weight. A person needs to remember "calories in, calories out," and the more strenuous the activity, the more "calories out." It is also important if comparing oneself to a pro athlete that one hears more than just the height and weight with respect to the athlete but also realizes the physical condition of the pro athlete and the possible contributing factors justifying a pro athletes weight.

IF YOU ARE OVERWEIGHT...

YOU ARE NOT:

"LARGE"

YOU ARE NOT:

A "PLUS SIZE"

YOU ARE NOT:

"FLUFFY"

YOU ARE FAT!

SO GO AHEAD, EAT THAT ENTIRE PIZZA, YOU PIG!

REMEMBER!!!!!!! IF YOU ARE FAT IT IS BECAUSE OF ONE OR MORE OF THE FOLLOWING:

You are lazy and inactive

You lack any discipline or self-control with respect to food and drink

You are apathetic with respect to your physical condition…. You don't give a damn.

Chapter Eight

PHYSICAL HEALTH

IF YOU ARE AN OVERLY FAT Person, if there is one reason above all else to change your lifestyle and lose that disgusting weight, it is for the reason of health. If you can't seem to want to do it for yourself then do it for a loved one, a spouse, your children or grand children, your girlfriend or boyfriend, because, believe it or not, your family would probably like you to be around for a while. And it is almost impossible to argue against the overwhelming evidence that connects obesity to an alarming number of health issues. So, if you're obese, are you so self-centered that you don't care if your children are devastated by your heart attack because you lack the self-discipline or self respect or general desire necessary to maintain some semblance of normalcy? If you are obese and are not doing something to change your life; then that means you don't care about yourself or your loved ones. And then my friend, I feel extremely sorry for you.

Let's summarize the various physical and mental ailments that go with being an Overly Fat Person. I will touch on them briefly here and then go into more detail with regard to specifics a little further on. There is the issue with heart disease, stroke and heart rhythm problems. There is the problem with the increased risk of diabetes and all the diseases and ailments that accompany diabetes. How about the added stress on bones, muscles, joints and tendons? Or, let me see, how about the effect fat has on the brain and how being fat makes the brain age faster? Or, how about the mental issues of depression or lack of self-image due to being fat? And there is much evidence that being obese increases the risk of many types of cancer.

HEART DISEASE AND STROKE

IF BEING A OFP AND HAVING to look at yourself in the mirror isn't disgusting enough to get you to do something about your blubber then maybe dying young due to heart disease or stroke might do the trick. Or if not dying, how about having a stroke due to your obesity and having to spend the rest of your life paralyzed or having diminished mental capacity? Sound nice? Consider the following from various articles/experts!

From the article Obesity and Heart Failure by Richard N. Fogoros, M.D. which can be read in its entirety on About.com Health and Disease

> Dateline: August 5, 2002
>
> "Doctors have suspected for a long time that overweight patients appear to have an increased risk of developing heart failure, but most believed that the heart failure resulted from the diabetes, high blood pressure and coronary artery disease associated with obesity. Now, however, a new study - published in the August 1 issue of the *New England Journal of Medicine* - shows that obesity itself (and not just the associated medical conditions) can lead to heart failure. "

Furthermore, the study shows that even excess body weight - in people who are not considered obese - substantially increases the risk of heart failure. " And thus this body weight can actually decrease an individuals life expectancy. The spare tire or love handles that so many individuals have is additionally harmful in that it can lead to harmful blood sugar levels and increased blood pressure. This condition of elevated blood glucose, hypertension and obesity is known in the medical community as the metabolic syndrome which over time can lead to diabetes and all of its harmful physical conditions.

And lastly, to my joy, the article concludes...

"The first step should be to increase activity and decrease caloric intake. Regular exercise will improve some of the metabolic problems associated with obesity but often aren't enough. Ask your doctor for more information and use the resources available on Livestrong. com."

The last paragraph is interesting isn't it? Gee, increase activity and cutting calories... what a novel idea! It's almost as if keeping one's weight respectable and increasing the likelyhood of good health is almost within one's reach. Of course, fat people would have to stop the rationalizing and actually utilize some self-control. How terrible!

The following information is even more interesting and every woman in the nation should be aware of these now common known associations with respect to obesity and pregancy. I have actually included a chapter in this book on pregnacy but the chapter deals more with womens attitudes and mental state as opposed to any health ramifications. But following is just a sample of what some research regarding the connection between obesity and pregancy can discover. And if you are a fat woman considering becoming pregnant you owe it to yourself, your spouse and your unborn child to consider your body weight before becoming pregnant.

Don't believe me? Consider this from My Pregnacyguide.com

"Did you know that gaining more than the recommended amount of weight during pregnancy also puts you at risk for being overweight several years after pregnancy?"

And not only does this negatively impact the obese/OFP mother but it negatively impacts the baby.

Further Mypregnancyguide.com states,

"The best thing you can do for yourself and the health of your unborn child is maintain a healthy weight prior to becoming pregnant."

Gee, what do you know! Maybe the women in our society should actually be at a "normal" body weight before they become pregnant. I never would have guessed it!!!!!!

This information comes from an article by Beverley Brooke, visit http://www.pregnancy-weight-loss.com for more on obesity and pregnancy

Do you think that it is just Heart Disease, Strokes and complications during pregnancy that should be cause for concern? Think again! How about the link between being overweight and cancer? And if you thought that my definition of an Overly Fat Person (OFP) was silly not being based on a BMI or something more objectively measured read excerpts from a very interesting article.

It is very interesting, is it not that (Epidemiology, September 2009) has this to say with respect to being over weight and the physical health relationship.

> "Your pants size might help gauge your risk of developing certain cancers, regardless of how much you actually weigh, Dutch researchers report. "

This increase in pants size relates to "intra-abdominal fat" and can lead to increased risks of type two diabetes, high blood pressure and heart disease.

In conclusion, the links to obesity and health issues are irrefutable. So if someone is a rational thinking human being how does this person justify putting him or herself in a condition such as being obese? How does a person literally play Russian roulette with their health? How does a person not think about the consequences of not only oneself but of their family? Does an obese person think of their family? Does an obese individual consider what it would be like for their children not to have a mother or father simply because they as obese individuals lack the self-discipline to control themselves with respect to food and drink?

IF YOU ARE OVERWEIGHT

YOU ARE NOT:

"PUDGEY"

YOU ARE NOT:

"BOUNCY"

YOU ARE NOT:

"BIG AND JOLLY"

YOU ARE FAT!

YOU ARE FAT !

REMEMBER!!!!!!! IF YOU ARE FAT IT IS BECAUSE OF ONE OR MORE OF THE FOLLOWING:

You are lazy and inactive

You lack any discipline or self-control with respect to food and drink

You are apathetic with respect to your physical condition…. You don't give a damn.

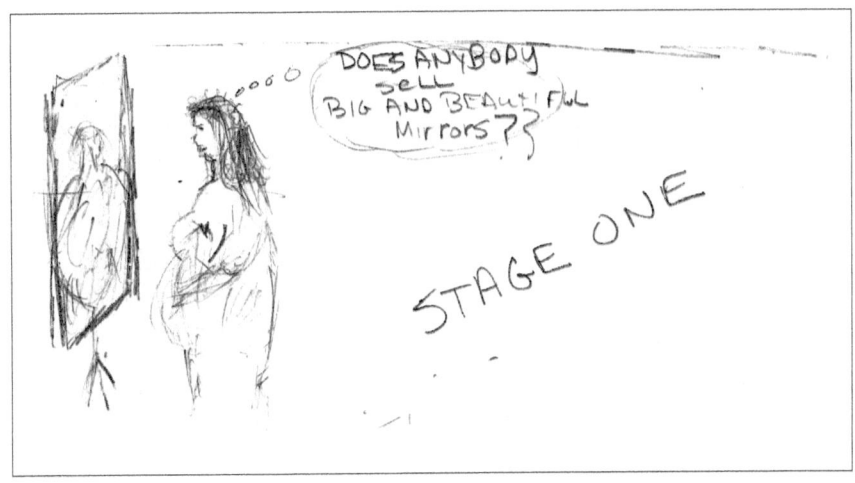

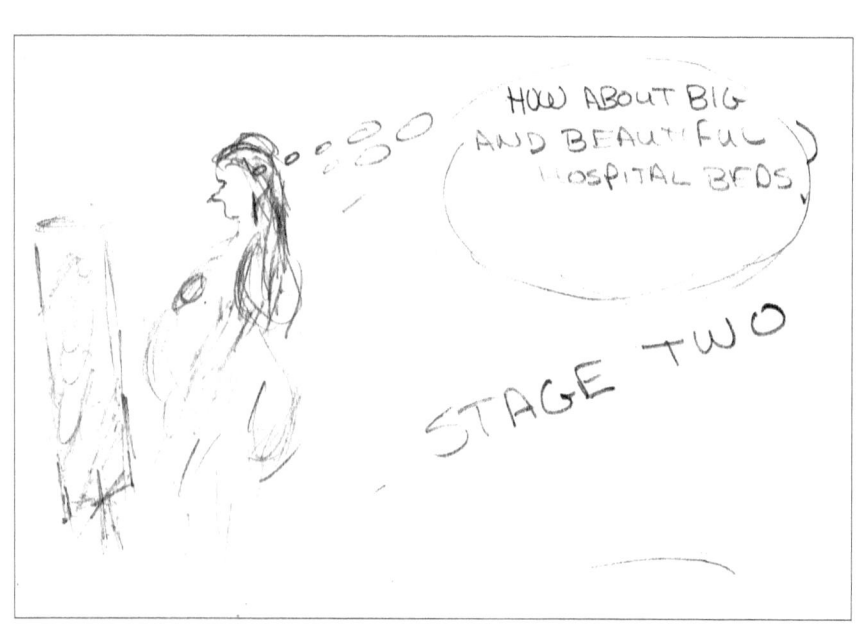

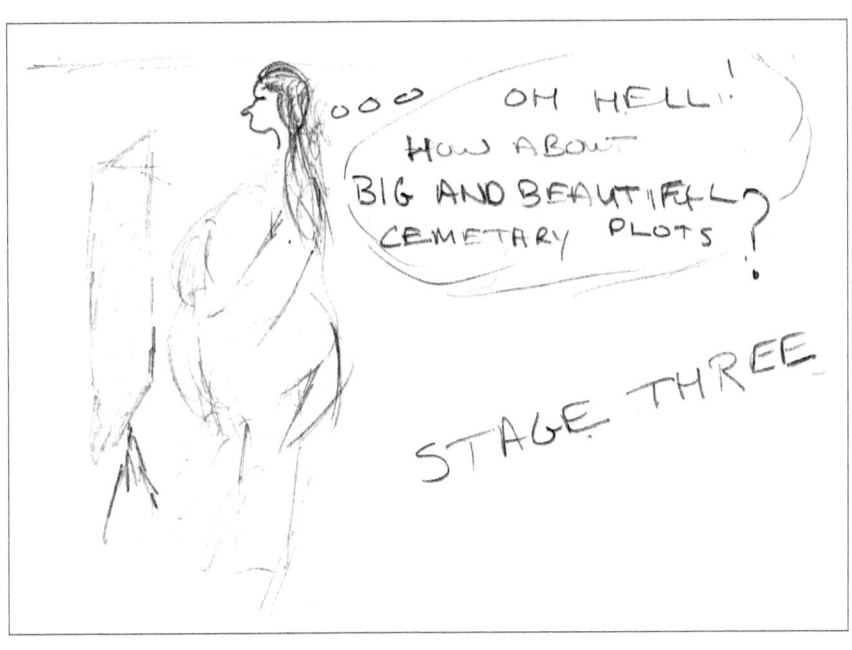

Chapter Nine

MENTAL HEALTH

IT SHOULD SEEM OBVIOUS TO EVERYONE that being "normal" and not a Overly Fat Person would help an individual with respect to their mental and physical "well being." But with so many people being fat and seemingly not giving a damn about their condition this must not be the case. So with that being said, let's explore why not being an OFP is beneficial in regard to your mental state of mind.

Let's take some obvious scenarios. The mirror! Every time you get out of the shower or put on your clothes you probably look at a mirror. If you don't you should because you need to be aware not only how your body feels but how your body appears. So let's suppose you are an OFP and you've just taken a shower. You are naked and as you step out of the shower you look in the mirror. Now don't try to tell me that if you weren't so fat that it would be a much more enjoyable experience! Don't try to tell me that if you could be in good physical condition that when exiting the showing and glancing in the mirror you wouldn't feel better about yourself!

Take another scenario, how about when people are about to have sex? Don't you think that people who are normal, who are fit, are more comfortable mentally then people who are fat and disgusting? Plus, people who are in better shape tend to perform better than those who are obese. And of course performing better is going to put a person in a much better mental state of mind for both themselves and their partner.

As one can easily see there is a strong relationship between an individuals physical condition and how they mentally perceive themselves. If a person is fat and gets out of the tub and sees themselves naked in the mirror, then unless they have been fooled by the "oh it's natural" crowd that doesn't understand the concept of self-discipline or accountability, they will not be in the greatest of mental states.

Another aspect of the mental health relationship to obesity is that typical activities that help individuals avoid becoming obese and activities that help people lose weight can have mental health benefits. For example, talk to people who love to run or play tennis or participate in other sports. Why do they participate in these endeavors? Do you think it is because they have dreams of turning pro? Well, maybe for the teenagers and young adults there are pipe dreams of stardom; but for most it is because they like the activities. And while individuals are engaged in these activities, and even after the fact, these activities make them feel better! These activities, at least for many of them, are a great way to increase mental health. From reducing stress to "feeling those endorphins kick in" to just strictly being entertainment, these endeavors increase in a positive way mental health. And these activities that people enjoy, through the burning of calories and of not eating (it's pretty difficult to eat a hot dog and play full court basketball or jog), help individuals control their weight.

The previous examples relate to an emphasis on mental well being due to physical appearance and physical fitness. The mirror and sex examples focused more on comfort, confidence and perception of ones self; with I guess, the obvious performance factor coming (no pun intended) into play with sex. But, like covered in the Health Chapter of this book, there is the physical health aspect of well-being. The chances of being healthy are much greater if your not obese! In fact, one could put forth a strong argument that if you are fat you are not healthy. So let's just say that if you are not fat or overtly obese you have better odds of not having chronic or acute symptoms of a disease or illness. And who can say they would not have a better mental outlook if they were not burdened with pain or illness? This is physical well being affecting your mental well-being.

There is also going to be the mentally uplifting effect related to the fact that the better an individual feels about themselves the happier, more content and the more self-confident that individual will be. This will lead to positive effects for individuals such as increased productivity at work, playing more with their children or maybe even their pets, and possibly having more friends all just because of the improved mental feeling related to not being overweight or extremely obese.

So in conclusion, it is obvious there is a connection, or should we say, relationship, between a person's physical state and their mental state. All those bleeding heart, Fat Sympathizers who are, maybe even without the realization of the fact, condoning the condition of obesity, have much to do with this obesity problem. But in the end, a person must have some accountability. An individual, with respect to obesity, IS in control of their destiny. And even though the "Fat Sympathizers" are, with their attitudes and actions toward obese people, "condoning" the condition of obesity and putting individuals in our great nation at a much higher risk of everything from heart disease, diabetes, strokes, certain cancers, etc., **we as a nation of great individualism must remain accountable!**

IF YOU ARE OVERWEIGHT

YOU ARE NOT:

"HEAVY"

YOU ARE NOT:

"FULL FIGURED"

YOU ARE NOT:

"WEIGHT CHALLENGED"

YOU ARE NOT:

"CHUBBY"

YOU ARE FAT!

AND YOU ARE RESPONSIBLE!

REMEMBER!!!!!!! IF YOU ARE FAT IT IS BECAUSE OF ONE OR MORE OF THE FOLLOWING:

You are lazy and inactive

You lack any discipline or self-control with respect to food and drink

You are apathetic with respect to your physical condition.... You don't give a damn.

Chapter Ten

ADVANTAGES TO LOSING WEIGHT- BEING NORMAL

THERE ARE MANY ADVANTAGES TO LOSING unnecessary weight beside the basic physical and mental health aspects. This chapter takes a closer look at some of the advantages an individual will reap by losing excess body weight. And for those of you reading who are not overweight these reasons are a great incentive to remain "Normal."

ACTIVITIES/SPORTS

ONE OF THE FIRST THINGS THAT come to my mind with respect to losing unwanted weight relates to sporting activities. Having participated in many, many different sports myself it is easy to relate the advantages of being at a good body weight for that specific sport.

RUNNING

I'D LIKE TO FIRST HAVE YOU consider running. The ability to run at your greatest potential is relevant to many sports. Running itself is one of the most basic of all sports and being at a good weight for your preferred distance is of supreme importance if you're to reach your ultimate potential as a runner. Now, this weight factor should seem obvious to most runners, but in my experience with other runners, especially recreational runners, it is a factor that is often overlooked or, surprise, surprise, rationalized. And contributing to this weight factor is that some recreational runners and joggers really have no idea of what a good body weight is for distance running or even sprinting. These individuals who run should do some reading on the subject of ideal body weights for runners. And it would also be very beneficial for the average runner to take a look at some elite runners with particular attention paid to these elite runners physiques. You would think with Americans being enamored with quick fixes that any distance runner/jogger would relish, in a relatively painless manner and over a relative brief amount of time, improving their times for their respective distance. But no! The biggest and most often heard excuse is that a runner has tried lowering their body weight but they feel weak and their times slow down. Or there is the (especially among men) "I don't want to lose any muscle" rationale. But these runners/joggers problem is that, like most of our society, they look "short term." So what if your long runs are slower when you are losing the weight? So what if you feel a little more tired when running hills or doing intervals! For heavens sake, think about 6 months down the road, not just your daily run! And so you runners/joggers, not only will your times improve after the weight loss, but you will be putting far less stress on your feet, knees, legs and back thus reducing the risk of injury! Geezzz, lose the weight.

Running is just one example of a sport where being at a good body weight is beneficial. You can take almost any sport that has some aerobic/cardio aspect and an Overly Fat Person can improve their performance significantly by weight reduction. You guys and gals out there who play basketball; if you are overweight now don't you think the game would be easy if you lost the excess baggage? How about you tennis players? How about you bikers?

Now let's take a look at some other activities to which being at a normal body weight is beneficial.

INTOXICATION

ANOTHER ADVANTAGE TO LOSING WEIGHT IS that it is much easier and cost effective to become intoxicated (yes, I think of everything!). The lower your body weight the less you will need to drink to feel a real good buzz. This also has obvious ramifications with respect to cost savings, as having to drink less to feel good requires less alcohol.

SEX

YOU WILL LOOK MORE ATTRACTIVE TO the opposite sex....oh yeah... or the same sex, depending on your preference (See, sometimes I can be Politically Correct) if you are not obese. And of course if you are not overweight you are likely to have more endurance, which if both partners are enjoying themselves, is a good thing.

GENERAL ACTIVITY

YOU WILL MORE THAN LIKELY BE more active if you are not overweight, as everything you do will take less effort. And when activities tire you less you will be more likely to participate in these activities for longer periods of time and more frequently. This is actually a GOOD "Catch-22."

SAVING MONEY

ONE OF THE GREAT BENEFITS OF losing weight is that you will be eating less, consequently, if you are eating the same foods but just less quantity, you will save money on your grocery bill.

OTHER REASONS TO LOSE WEIGHT

*I MUST EXPLAIN SOMETHING NOW SO as to not lose credibility with respect to the serious nature of this book; to those who can't distinguish between when someone is serious or not, **some** of the below reasons to lose weight need to be taken somewhat lightly!*

You will fit more comfortably in airline and theater seats if you are not overweight.

You will get better gas mileage in your car, especially if previously you were extremely overweight.

Your wife and children will respect you more if you are normal. Your family will be more proud of you. When you pick-up your children at school they will no longer be embarrassed by your size. Plus, you'll be setting a good example for your children as far as a healthier lifestyle is concerned. This hopefully will prevent your children from having weight issues now or in the future.

You will receive many, many compliments from impressed co-workers if you lose weight thus improving your mental outlook and maybe even increasing promotional opportunities at work.

Your dog will love you more! (Well, maybe!)

You won't be embarrassed about your clothes or waist size if you drop the excess weight.

If you are not overweight you won't have to worry when at the beach about Greenpeace trying to save you after mistaking you for a whale.

It will be easier to tie your shoes and cut your toenails if you are not an Overly Fat Person.

It will be easier to wipe yourself after bowel movements if you are not extremely overweight. Now don't laugh. I remember seeing a special on television about Sumo Wrestlers in Japan. According to this special, it sounded as if wiping oneself is difficult when you are the size of a typical Sumo Wrestler. And because of this difficulty factor when wiping one's ass, the Rookie or Novice Sumo Wrestlers sometimes have the responsibility of wiping the senior Sumo's you know what. So it must be easier to wipe if you are thin.

You will be cooler in the hot summer months if you are of normal body weight. Of course the negative side of this is that in the colder months you may have to dress warmer. But then again, it is much easier to dress warmer; you can only take off so much in the way of clothes when it's hot…. Once you're down to your skin you have pretty much reached your limit.

Already mentioned in other chapters of this book, but when you are lighter there is much less weight related stress and impact on many areas of your body. Even your back will feel better with substantial weight loss.

Fat person jokes might not offend you so much if you were to take off some pounds!

If more Americans lost weight there would be less chance that the planet will be thrown out of orbit due to severe tilting of the earth due to the heaviness of America.

You will be less likely to break furniture when sitting down if you are not obese.

If you fall on your pet you will be less likely to kill the poor thing if you weigh less.

It will be easier to walk more softly and more quietly if you are lighter on your feet. This can save wear and tear on the carpet, let your spouse sleep more soundly when you are walking about, keep water in puddles calm so as neighbors won't think Godzilla or T-Rex is approaching, and it will be easier on your arches if you are not fat.

If you are incapacitated or injured it will be easier for rescue personnel to pull you to safety if you have lost weight.

Just think of the natural resources that could be saved if all Americans were to lose weight, requiring smaller clothes sizes and thus less fabric!

There is less danger of the elevator you are on of being overloaded poundage wise if you are not an Overly Fat Person.

If you are not overweight you present less of a target for a terrorist or a sniper.

So after reading this chapter about all the fantastic benefits to being of normal body weight, why would anyone wish to remain fat?

IF YOU ARE OVERWEIGHT

YOU ARE NOT:

"JUST PACKIN' ON THE POUNDS"

YOU ARE NOT:

"GETTING OLDER"

YOU ARE NOT:

"A LARGE SIZED PERSON"

YOU ARE FAT!

YOU ARE FAT AND YOU NEED TO DO SOMETHING ABOUT IT!

REMEMBER!!!!!!! IF YOU ARE FAT IT IS BECAUSE OF ONE OR MORE OF THE FOLLOWING:

You are lazy and inactive

You lack any discipline or self-control with respect to food and drink

You are apathetic with respect to your physical condition…. You don't give a damn.

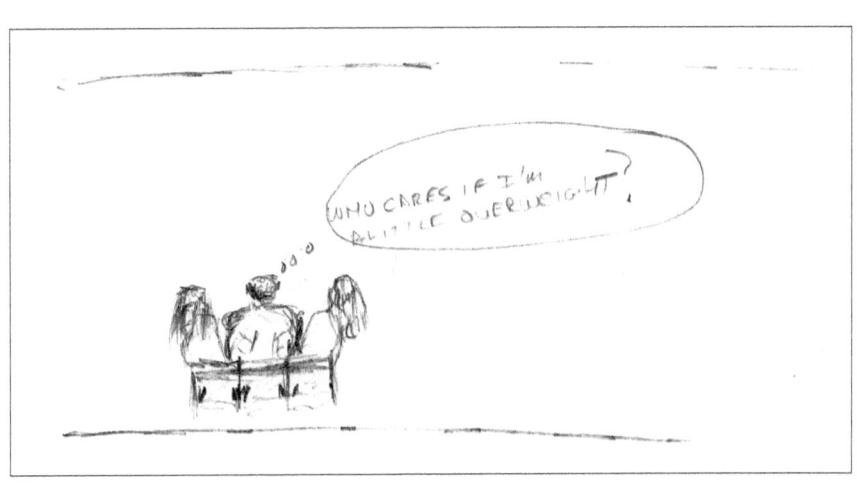

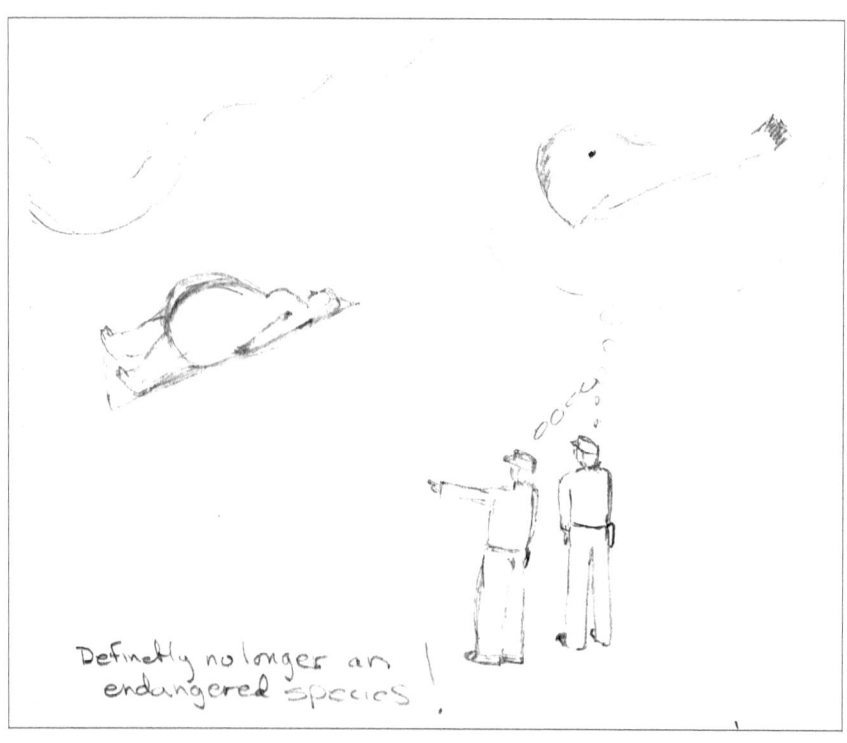

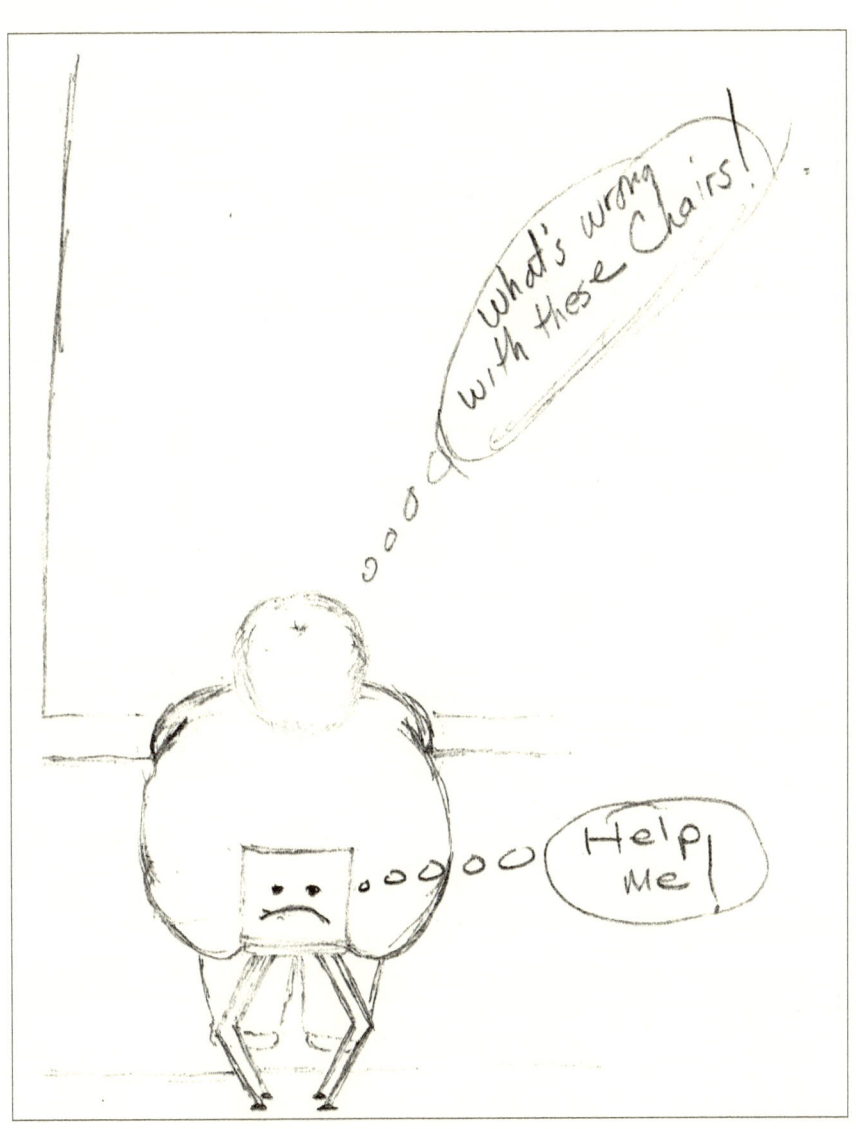

Chapter Eleven

POLLUTION

WELL NOW, ALL YOU READERS WHO hate every word that I have written so far... wait till you get a load of what's in this chapter!

With all the talk of pollution these days, with everything from air pollution causing global warming to plastics in our landfills to pesticides in our drinking water, there is one form of pollution that is not often discussed. There is one form of pollution that is "hush, hush." There is one form of pollution that we dare not discuss! So some people just look the other way as opposed to mentioning this pollution. Some people notice the pollution and try to rationalize. While still others might just chuckle and are thinking "I guess there is not much we can do about it." And worse yet, others don't even notice the pollution because this form of pollution is becoming commonplace in our nation. What is this form of pollution that is threatening our nation? What is this form of pollution that makes many of us sick? What is this devious form of pollution that makes many of us disgusted when we visit our nation's scenic rivers and beaches on glorious summer days? What is this form of pollution that can ruin our visits to the pool or spa? This pollution can even affect us when visiting our favorite restaurants or when shopping. What is this form of pollution?????? It is Visual Pollution. It is the visual pollution caused by Overly Fat People (OFP).

Laugh if you want. But let me ask you something; let me ask those of you who have gone to the beach on a hot summers day to imagine this scenario. As you are walking down the beach or maybe even just relaxing on a towel or in a beach chair, you happen to notice something large approaching. What could this be, a dying whale or Sea Lion having been washed ashore? What could this moving large object be? As this object nears it becomes somewhat apparent that it is too small for a whale, at least too small for an adult male whale. But maybe it still could be a Sea Lion. But no, as the object approaches you notice that it is a human being. But how could this be? How could a human be so large? As the object/human comes nearer you begin to realize that this person is just extremely obese. And now, as the person closes in, your curiosity and wonderment turns to repulsion and disgust. You have suddenly lost that desire for the last bite of your sandwich as you watch the belly rolls jostle up and down and from side to side on this Overly Fat Person. It is disgusting and beyond comprehension that for some reason this obese individual has decided that wearing a bikini is their right as a U.S. Citizen. (Is it your right as a U.S. citizen to urinate in public, display porn in public, etc. etc.?) You are amazed at how this person walks as if they are actually proud of their obese, disfigured, disgusting body. That, my friends, is the visual pollution caused by overweight and obese individuals. And this form of pollution is mentally harming our nation.

So do you think this obesity of humans is not visual pollution, let me ask you this; how pleasant is it when at work during the summer, in a nice air-conditioned office, and low and behold along comes some 300-pound lady wearing a tight dress thinking she is gods gift to humanity? Does this not disgust you? Does the sight of this obese individual not revolt you? And are you not simultaneously wondering why this person has let their body deteriorate to such an extent? And why on God's earth does this individual, and others like her, actually appear to be "showing off" their body in some form of sick, perverse exhibitionism? This is Visual Pollution! And we, the normal portion of the population, should not have to tolerate such disgusting displays of fat!

Now, not to be redundant, but let me reiterate that being fat is unlike having a not so cute face. We can't do much about our faces... unless we are wealthy and have idolized Michael Jackson's plastic surgery philosophy.... But we can control our weight. So don't start down the path of feeling sorry for these visual polluters. People need to take responsibility for their actions (stuffing their faces with food and drink) and also think of others. Does that fat 300 pound women in her revealing dress ever stop to think that maybe she is not attractive? She should! Does that fat woman not only realize that when she wantonly displays her obesity she is not attractive but actually repulsive! She should!

What has become of our nation that such examples of repulsively fat people causing visual pollution are becoming commonplace? Why do people who are overly fat not realize that their visual appearance is repulsive? Why do normal people put up with the visual pollution in their everyday lives? Why do some people, even the individuals who are not obese, often view fat disgusting people as NOT fat and disgusting? It is the answer to these questions that is helping cause the obesity epidemic that permeates our American society.

This acceptance and lack of acknowledgement by the general public with respect to the repulsiveness of obese people is due to a few very important factors. First and foremost is the "Political Correctness" factor. Political Correctness is a very important reason that OFP's can get away with disgusting others. Heaven forbid if we, as non-obese normal people, ever say something negative with respect to these Overly Fat People. Our society feels we should, as normal people, just accept these fat slobs. We should accept these fat individuals as people who are just cursed by nature; that is how we have recently been conditioned to think by political correctness. And what has this political correctness caused? It has been one of the chief contributing factors responsible for our nations fat epidemic. Hey, maybe we should also be Politically Correct and basically condone smoking, alcoholism and deviant behavior!

Another group of people who contribute to visual pollution and our nations fat epidemic are the "Fat Sympathizers." These "Fat Sympathizers" view/perspective, that we as a culture should empathize with fat people, allows fat and obese individuals a way to rationalize their condition and falsely feel proud about their disgustingly repulsive bodies as if it were natural for them to be in this state of obesity. Heaven forbid we disrespect fat slobs…. "It is just the way nature intended these obese people to look." "Oh, these poor overweight, plump and big and beautiful people, they have no control over their bodies; let's respect them and make them feel normal." Bullshit to you "Fat Sympathizers" who have this attitude that being fat is normal. To Hell with all you "Fat Sympathizers," you that just compound the problem of our nations obesity epidemic.

And, in an indirect fashion, there are actually entities in our nation that like the fact that so many in our population are fat and obese. So what entities care about people remaining obese? Just consider all the companies that profit from the quick fix attitude of the American public. Think about the diet pill manufacturers and the profits they would lose if everyone just consumed less calories and lost weight? Of course they feel safe because most fat Americans don't have the self-control or discipline to just EAT LESS!!!!! Also, don't you think the diet pill manufacturers know that the average person who losses weight with their diet pills will gain the weight right back after discontinuing pill usage because these pill poppers won't change their eating habits and lifestyle? How about the clothes manufacturers who specialize in apparel for the overly obese? The list goes on an on. And this list, in an indirect fashion, does contribute to our nations visual pollution.

So Guys, don't expect to see only "hot babes" on the beach in the near future. Just expect to see those proud women with the roles of fat bouncing near and far between sections of her bikini stroll down the beach as if they were hot commodities; all the while you somehow resist the urge to puke. And Gals, the "hunks" will be few and far between! You Gals better get used to seeing that beer bellied guy without a shirt walk around exposing his gut as if were some grotesque obtuse phallic symbol; and how he is somehow oblivious to the disgust of all who must watch him parade around.

BUT HEY, THOSE AREN'T FAT PEOPLE; THEY ARE "BIG AND BEAUTIFUL" PEOPLE!

IF YOU ARE OVERWEIGHT...

YOU ARE NOT:

"HEAVY"

YOU ARE NOT:

"FULL FIGURED"

YOU ARE NOT:

"CHUBBY"

YOU ARE FAT!

YOU ARE A SORRY EXCUSE FOR A HUMAN- CHANGE!

REMEMBER!!!!!!! IF YOU ARE FAT IT IS BECAUSE OF ONE OR MORE OF THE FOLLOWING:

You are lazy and inactive

You lack any discipline or self-control with respect to food and drink

You are apathetic with respect to your physical condition…. You don't give a damn.

Chapter Twelve

DIETS -WEIGHT LOSS

IN THIS CHAPTER I COVER DIETS (obviously) and I also put in my two cents worth about diets, fasting, special food programs and also add some tips on ways individuals can lose weight. Many of these tips are seen and heard everywhere and are commonplace methods to lose weight in our society. But some of the tips I offer may not be known by readers and anything that can maybe help someone lose weight is a good thing, right? But before we get to that good stuff I would like to discuss diets.

(I would like to note here that this chapter and the chapter on Competitiveness (some might argue the entire book) are not the best-written chapters in literary history. Please don't let the lack of organization or the writing ability of the Author influence whether or not the reader believes the points presented are valid or useful.)

So what do you do if you are an Overly Fat Person? Well, suck it up so to speak and lose weight. Nobody cares (well, I guess lots of people who stand to make money care) how you do it; just lose weight. The ultimate key for long-term success is going to be changing your lifestyle with respect to food and activity. We all deep down inside know this fact about needing to change an individuals lifestyle to lose weight long term but most don't want to face this fact because it involves activity, self-disciple and actually taking pride in one's body.

So to lose all that weight that you have accumulated over the years will take some doing. The basic answer of what to do involves lowering caloric intake, burning more calories or both. This chapter discusses lowering your caloric intake. And there are various approaches to lowering your caloric intake. For example, you can attempt to lose the weight quickly; thus going on a "diet." Or, you can lose the weight in a gradual manner by a lifestyle change, or you can diet and then change your lifestyle. This chapter discusses the pros and cons to the quick loss of weight; also known as the successful diet.

DIETS

So you are going to go on a diet. Your problem will be solved. In no time at all you will be transformed into a fit and trim model like individual. And then of course you will be able to revert back to eating anything and everything you want. Wrong, but like I have stated, most people are aware of this fact but just don't want to face it. Boy, they think, once you've lost that weight you can begin living again. Right? Maybe! And this is where the controversy begins. Do diets work?

DO DIETS WORK?

You hear people discussing diets all the time. People are talking about which diet is best, which diets they've tried, etc., etc. But the big question is do diets work? And you will hear my strong opinions with respect to whether or not diets do indeed work or not. But the answer to the question in large part depends on your definition of "work." In my mind, from what I have personally experienced and what I have seen from countless people on diets, diets do indeed work! They work in that while you are on the diet you do indeed lose weight. And really, that is all the diets claim to do, help you lose weight while you are on the diet! But somehow there are people out there in the real world who expect diets to be some panacea for people who have major issues with respect to their personality. And these personality issues are why these individuals gained weight and had to go on a diet in the first place. If you haven't guessed already, the issues are activity, self-discipline and apathy. These issues of character/personality traits are difficult to permanently resolve. Case in point, the fact that most people lose weight on a diet yet will ultimately gain this weight back after returning to their previous habits/lifestyle, the lifestyle that caused them to gain all the extra weight in the first place. But again, the answer to the question of do diets work and the answer is YES, diets do work.

Now, let's delve into some specific diet programs and how they work. And let's reflect on why people use diets and why, although they will more then likely get results, once they go off the diet (not to be overly redundant here but…) and revert back to their old ways they will gain all the weight back.

The basic premise of "calories in, calories out" is true. And this is how the majority of diets aid in an individuals weight loss, the diets reduce an individual's caloric intake. Even the diets that are meal plans, even though these companies insist their plans work because of scientifically developed formulas/recipes that are an ideal balance of the just right type of carbohydrates and the proper balance of just the right proteins and just the right vitamins and minerals, and just the right… Well, upon closer inspection you will notice these meals are very low in calories. Hmmmm. "Calories in, calories out," what a novel concept (In a later chapter I delve into why these meal plan companies and others want to deceive you. Hint, $$$$). But diets do work! But also it doesn't take a rocket scientist to realize that if an individual loses the weight by caloric reduction and increased activity…. burning calories, limiting calories, thus losing weight… that once you return to your old habits you will gain the weight back. But, the diet did indeed work; it reduced your body weight.

A person might counter my backing of the "calories in, calories" out belief with, "I went on a low carb diet and I lost 20 pounds." But I bet when this person was eliminating the carbohydrates from their diet they were not replacing the calories in the carbohydrates with a like amount of calories from say, protein. For example, an individual dines out a lot and starts a low carb diet. At all their meals they stop eating anything high in carbs. This individual over the course of time loses 20 pounds and proclaims the carb diet a success! But this individual lost the weight because he/she did not eat the rice or the bread or the potato … AND… did not replace the rice, bread, or potato calories with any other calories. Thus, all this individual did was lower their caloric intake. Oh Well!

So what should a person do? What is the ultimate answer? The answer is already out there and many experts (dietitians, fitness guru's, nutritionists, etc.) have already told you repeatedly the answer. But our society doesn't like their answer. Because their answer involves more then a quick fix. Their answer involves some discipline and self-control. Gee, what a thought; discipline and self-control in a person's life; and for what? Just to look good, be in better health, feel better physically and emotionally and on and on. That's quite a sacrifice; you bet your life it is! And that may be literal (see Physical Health chapter).

LARGEST PROBLEMS WITH DIETING:

So you have decided to diet. Let's discuss the problems with diets and leave out of the discussion, the already mentioned 100 times previously, the fact that after the diet you can't just return to the previous lifestyle that caused you to be an Overly Fat Person in the first place.

And I guess it would be somewhat pertinent to before giving my input on diets to mention that I have experience losing weight. I have been as heavy as 215 pounds and as light as 154 pounds. At 215 I was definitely not all fat as I was running and lifting weights. I could bench over 20 reps of 225 pounds at the 215-pound body weight so I certainly had some muscle. However, I also had a larger waist size than I wanted to go along with my muscular upper body. Therefore when I lost weight, not only did I lose some muscle but also I did indeed lose a significant amount of body fat. I should also mention that when I weighed 154 pounds I was not weight lifting, I was running over 60 miles per week and I was also dieting. Needless to say, that was not very healthy and it didn't last long as became weak and susceptible to injuries. So I mention this to you as a reader to make you aware of the fact that I can practice what I preach and I do have vast knowledge of exercise and fitness programs along with having researched and been on various diets. My favorite diet by the way was my "Beer" diet; not the healthiest diet but it was the most enjoyable. And the beer diet definitely supports my utmost confidence in the "calories in, calories out," theories and principles.

Now, back to diets. In the author's opinion, the biggest problem with going on a typical "diet" is the fact that you are always thinking about your diet. Sound strange? Well, not really. When you are on a diet what, besides the overall diet and objective, are you thinking? You are always thinking about FOOD. Should I eat this food or should I eat that food. What should I eat for breakfast? How about lunch? And what are my plans for dinner? Most people on a diet are constantly thinking about food when they are on that diet. The key to losing weight is not to have food the primary focus in your life. Now, not that any of you have ever heard of the expression, " Eat to live, don't live to eat" but if you can incorporate that belief system into your life than you will have it made. How do you do this? How do you eat to live as opposed to living to eat? Well, for one, a person can still just eat the same foods but just eat less of those foods. That way the person is not constantly thinking about what to eat or what not to eat. The person just eats as normal with the exception of serving/portion size.

WHICH DIETS?

So EVEN THOUGH IT MAY APPEAR I am not for so-called "diets," in fact I am, well kinda. After the diet you must change your life style. But if you don't do something a little drastic initially, it will take you forever to lose much weight. Thus, you will become discouraged and possibly return to the lifestyle that caused you to become as obese as you are now.

So which diets do I recommend? What did the "kinda" in the previous paragraph mean? Well, if you have found a diet that works for you great! By all means use that diet. But keep in mind that after the diet you must by all means NOT revert back to your old eating habits and lifestyle.

SAVE YOUR MONEY

But, ALTHOUGH I BELIEVE IN DIETS, my view on promoted/ advertised and popular diets is that they can be a total waste of money. Think about it. On a diet you are reducing caloric intake; and maybe simultaneously increasing physical activity and thus also burning more calories. So why do you need to spend money on special foods or recipes or whatever. YOU DON'T!

An important point I would like to make with respect to diets and saving money deals with our societies gullibility to propaganda. Our nations public, although intelligent, is also extremely gullible. People will believe almost anyone who has supposed authority, anyone with a white doctors coat or named Milgram. This is especially true in times of economic hardship, mental depression and for that matter, being severely overweight. During these times of hardship the public will believe and trust anyone who promises utopia, is handsome and reads well from a teleprompter. It somehow is not significant to the gullible public that said individual attends a racist church, associates with unrepentant terrorists, and surrounds himself with self proclaimed communists and, for icing on the cake, tells us with disrespect that we should go cling to our Bibles and guns. This same gullibility is a partial reason so many fat people try the diet pills or plans, the special foods, the special supposedly unique exercise programs, etc. even though deep down they know that these gimmicks are not necessary and by just using self-discipline their problems would be solved and their money would be saved.

My basic premise is that a diet should SAVE YOU MONEY! You can lose a ton of weight.... Well, not literally, well yes literally if you are on one of those cable specials.... You can lose a lot of weight by just reducing your caloric intake and increasing physical activity. So eat less of what you are eating right now. It is pretty simple, yes? And of course, think of the money you will save. It may not go over well with all the diet pill manufacturers or the specialty food/ diet program companies out there; but why help make them rich?

If a person wanted. If a person had some self-discipline, above and beyond losing the weight by eating less, they could actually start some type of diet investment fund. All you have to do is calculate how much money you are saving each month by eating less and invest that money. Or, instead of saving the money, use the extra money as discretionary income and spend it on something that brings you enjoyment. NOT HIGH CALORIE FOOD.

FASTING:

I AM A FIRM BELIEVER THAT a short-lived neo-fast is greatly beneficial for most individuals. Now what I mean by a neo-fast is a fast that eliminates all foods but contains non-caloric beverages. The beverages can be water, which is the most common, or for individuals who may need a little "zip" for energy beverages can include black coffee or diet soda. I don't recommend the 'fasting' that incorporates certain ingredients that supposedly help your body eliminate certain unhealthy byproducts. I feel that because the instructions for this type of fasting that cleanses your system also state something to the extent that not only are you removing harmful byproducts but you are also eliminating beneficial bacteria and by-products. So then you must intake certain products to restore your bodies helpful bacteria and organisms. This sounds a little scary to me. Why not just keep it simple and simply fast? Besides, if you simply fast you are also saving money.

What might you ask are the benefits of fasting? I feel the most important reasons to fast be strictly psychological in nature. Fasting will make you realize that missing a meal or two will not literally kill you. Fasting will also help you understand better what true hunger feels like and discern true hunger from what are cravings or self programmed/conditional responses at certain times of the day relating to the consumption of food.

So what is hunger? Not many Americans truly know the feeling of hunger. I am sure none of us has or will ever experience the hunger associated with Stalingrad during the WWII siege. We will never know what or how the Donner Party felt on their unfortunate travels in the Sierra Nevada mountain range (talk about an eating disorder controversy). In my mind it is a joke that people go crazy with hunger when they miss a lunch. Give me a break! So, what a one or two day fast will do for you is make you aware of what is real (to a certain degree) hunger and what are just cravings.

Fasting will also toughen your mind. For instance, if you can go one or two days without any food, just think how easy it will be to live on 1500 calories a day! 1500 calories a day will be a feast! Fasting will force you to use self-discipline to achieve a goal, that of weight loss. But this increase of self-discipline is not only beneficial in terms of losing weight loss but also in other arenas of life. Increasing one's self discipline can improve an individual's performance at work, completing chores around the house, or with respect to sports or other activities.

FASTING-CARDIO/AEROBICS-HEALTHY FOOD

AN AMAZING THING WILL HAPPEN IF you incorporate fasting, intense cardio/aerobic activity, subsequent dieting and forcing yourself to eat **healthy** foods, even if just for a short period of time. A short period of time being defined as: a few weeks to a month, more or less. Suddenly, the foods that you thought tasted so good, well they now taste horrendous, and you wonder how you or anyone else could eat such disgusting food. You will take a bite of that sausage or piece of bacon, which smells so good, and probably want to spit it out. That pizza that you enjoyed so much while watching your favorite television program will suddenly seem so greasy and oily that you have to force yourself to eat a slice. That super dark micro beer that previously tasted so good will be replaced by a "light beer." A bite into your favorite candy bar may give you a big surprise! The candy bar that you loved so dearly previously will now not taste good at all and you will literally have to force yourself to finish the bar.

FAVORITE FOOD OR BEVERAGE DIET

BEFORE CLOSING THIS CHAPTER SOME OF you might be curious as to what in the world was my Beer Diet? And in describing my Beer Diet, one realizes that an individual can easily (and should) develop his or her own diet. My favorite diet, has and probably always will be, my Beer Diet. Do I need to say more? Well, I guess I probably need to explain. My Beer Diet was/is simply a small lunch (small being caloric related not food specific) followed by (in the evening) beer… much beer and some more beer and a small dinner. A couple of important items to note are that the important factor in the beer diet is total caloric intake for the day. So if I had a lunch of say, 500 calories, I figured I could have a dinner of at least 1000 calories and still lose weight based on the calories in, calories out formula. So if you do the math, if a light beer had approximately 100 calories I would use a formula dependent on how much beer I wish to drink that night. Typically I would down 4 to 6 beers and use the remaining calories on food. And by food, well, yes that sometimes was chips! One key factor in my Beer Diet, which allowed me to feel "full" and satisfied, sooner, was that I would have a few beers before eating. This drinking of the beer first accomplished two things; first, like mentioned, it made me feel full just as the old drinking a couple of glasses of water before eating trick. Second, drinking the beer on an empty stomach would let me feel much better, so to speak, in a short period of time. So, in addition to the fullness factor and thus feeling like eating less, there was the intoxication factor. I should also mention that I would not go to extremes with my beer diet if I were out in public due to the driving factor. More often then not I would basically do the George Thorogood, "*I drink Alone*" routine at home. Now that I have appeased MADD I guess I must next cope with AA; but so be it!

So as one can easily see… what is readily apparent… is that an individual can substitute the beer in my Beer Diet for any of their favorite food or drink. A person just needs to calculate total calories and keep these calories at a low level to be certain of losing weight. Also, by an individual using their favorite food or drink in their diet it helps tremendously with respect to reducing individual's cravings. And best yet, with this favorite food diet, one can lose weight and simultaneously have fun!

GET A LIFE!

WELL, ONE WAY TO "EAT TO live" is to get a life! Is food your only reason for living? Is it the only thing that gives you enjoyment in your life? Is your next meal all you think about during the day? If so then you are a "sad" individual. But don't feel bad; a large portion of our society is just like you! But ask yourself; don't you have family and friends? Do you not work or have social activities that can keep your mind occupied? Do you workout or have sporting activities that stimulate your body and mind? Do you like or enjoy sex? (And if you don't, maybe losing some weight will help, huh) Do you have hobbies that can keep your mind occupied and your hands busy?

A point I would like to make here because it seems to be an opportune time to do so is related to hobbies, friends, and general activities. This seems rather obvious but make sure your activities are not focused around food. And if food is present, use some self-control. Every time you see or are around food you don't have to eat till you can no longer eat anymore for fear of your stomach exploding. Also, change some of your habits that add on the additional calories. For instance, if you are going to a basketball game eat dinner before you go to the game. Then, once you arrive at the game, forgo the hotdogs, beer, (well, maybe not the beer) popcorn and other snacks that not only drive up the price of the evening but also add on those additional calories. Or, for that matter, if you have weak self-discipline, forgo your dinner and eat at the game. Just don't do both. Remember it is "calories in-calories out" (just like my Beer diet). Just don't give yourself the double whammy!

So an Overly Fat Person who wants to lose weight should try to become involved in activities that are not only healthy but also don't involve the obligatory over indulgence of food or beverage. As an example, I see guys in these laid back softball leagues where it would be fine if they just played softball (although not the most calorie burning activity, it sure is better than the sofa) but these individuals don't just play softball, they eat the most fatty and high caloric foods and beverages available. How is this type of softball going to help someone lose weight?

The key point in all of this to remember is to stay mentally or physically active or preoccupied. Then food will not be the focal point of your existence. Haven't you ever been so busy at work with something of the utmost importance that you actually forgot to have lunch? And by the way, because you missed lunch did you die? Did you have a mental breakdown? Did you lose 5 pounds of muscle? Of course you didn't die or have a mental breakdown or lose massive amounts of muscle just because you missed lunch. The more then obvious point here is that if you miss a meal you are not destroying your body. But back to the main point, I think it is easy for you to see that if you can maintain physical or mental activity you will eat less and the weight will come off.

TRICKS I HAVE USED TO LOSE WEIGHT

LIKE I HAVE MENTIONED, OVER THE years there has been a few instances when it became necessary for me to lose weight. As mentioned in the opening paragraph of this chapter some of my tricks have been used by millions of people. But there is the possibility that I have used some tricks with which people are not aware with respect to losing weight. So in the interest of a lighter America, here I go!

One of the best ways I have found to lose weight has been to become involved in a sport or activity. The important factor here is not so much that this sport or activity was something that burned calories, although that is more beneficial, but that the reason I participated in the activity or sport was that the activity was enjoyable. So the activity was not designed to lose calories but was **FUN**. This partaking in an activity that is fun is much different and much easier mentally then exercise with the sole purpose of losing weight. It is much easier mentally to spend two hours on a tennis court if you enjoy tennis than it is if you go on a 5-mile jog when the only reason for the jog is to burn calories… and deep down you detest jogging! So if there is some sport or activity you previously enjoyed but for whatever reason you stopped… then start again. And for you others who don't have an activity in your past that you enjoyed…. well, try something new. Get a life!

Depending on the individual's preferences almost any activity can be enjoyable and help in weight loss. I was fortunate enough to actually enjoy running, so until I developed OA in my right knee, I was able to lose much weight just by running 40 or more miles a week and simultaneously enjoy all the running. But seeing everyone is different, I will list just a few of the sports/activities that come to mind that a person might find enjoyable and aid in the reduction of a weight. Maybe one of these will strike a fancy with you. Some of these activities are much better at burning calories than others; but all of these activities are better than sitting on a couch eating chips and drinking beer.

ACTIVITIES:

Running
Sex
Swimming
Golf
Baseball and Softball
Basketball, full court or other
Hiking
Football
Tennis
Volleyball
Skateboarding
Motocross
Biking
Walking your dog
Playing with your pets
Yard-work
Gardening
Walking
Skating
Skiing
Water Polo
Bowling
Shopping in the Mall
Cleaning house
Martial Arts
Boxing
Wrestling

As you can see, the list is endless. Use your imagination to think of ways to burn calories and get your, you know what, off the couch. And keep in mind that you can burn more calories in a certain activity by just making the activity more intense. For instance, there is basketball and there is basketball. Playing Horse will not burn the same amount of calories as a full court game of basketball. There is tennis and there is tennis. Just going out on the court and rallying right to each other is not the same as playing a couple long sets with long points. Even yard work can be made more intense. For example, get rid of that loud, annoying leaf blower that probably bothers your neighbors to no end, but they are too polite to tell you, and use a leaf rake!

I know one activity, which most people should partake but don't. And this is striking because supposedly everyone loves his or her dog, right? Well, if you really love your dog you must allow the pet to actually have some exercise. Walking the dog is a great mental treat for your dog but it does little for keeping your dog in shape and healthy. SO, take your dog running or jogging with you! And seeing a run/jog for you may be intense, it is not very intense for your dog. Jogging, which is like a fast walk for your dog, is still not using the dogs fast twitch muscles (I guess this would be true for some breeds and not others,). So, because of this, make sure you let the dog run and jump. I do this by playing catch with my dog using a Frisbee. So my dog gets a two-mile jog about 5 times a week and also gets to run and jump for Frisbees everyday. I have also seen people that ride their bikes with their dog running alongside. I am not sure I am too keen on this because of safety concerns for both the rider and the dog. But if you have a safe place to ride and a very well trained dog then go for it. But the point is this, if you are playing with your dog or running with your dog the activity is mutually beneficial!

Another important aspect of an activity, which I touched upon previously, is that even if the activity is not strenuous, if the activity is mentally engaging the activity can be beneficial with respect to losing weight. How? Because, if an individual is mentally engaged with an enjoyable activity, more then likely this individual is not thinking about food. This is very important for not only dieting but for the lifestyle change that must take place after the diet.

EAT ONLY WHEN HUNGRY

ANOTHER TRICK I HAVE LEARNED.... OR more accurately, a principle; is to never eat when you are **not** hungry. Sounds simple right? Well, not really. We are conditioned to eat certain meals at certain times. We are told, "breakfast is the most important meal, and you must eat breakfast." Well, I am of the opinion that if you are not hungry, then don't eat. If you are not hungry in the morning then don't eat breakfast. Trust me, you won't die! Your body will tell you when you need to eat. The same, "when not hungry then don't eat," applies to any meal!

BEVERAGES

ANOTHER AREA TO WATCH WITH RESPECT to losing weight deals with beverages. A person should definitely take notice of the caloric content in the beverages they drink. By drinking just water it is amazing how many extra calories you can consume on food and yet still lose weight. People just don't realize the amount of calories in a glass of orange juice or in a regular soft drink (or in beer?).

In closing this chapter, the important things to remember are that you can lose weight by dieting, fasting and other tricks. You can also be saving money while you are losing weight just by reducing the amount of foods and beverages you presently consume. And finally, you can have pleasure while losing weight by just enjoying activities that are "FUN!"

-IF YOU ARE OVERWEIGHT…

YOU ARE NOT:

"WELL INSULATED"

YOU ARE NOT:

"CHUBBY"

YOU ARE NOT:

"WEIGHT CHALLENGED"

YOU ARE FAT!

YOU ARE RISKING YOUR HEALTH—MIGHT AS WELL SMOKE TOO!

REMEMBER!!!!!!! IF YOU ARE FAT IT IS BECAUSE OF ONE OR MORE OF THE FOLLOWING:

You are lazy and inactive

You lack any discipline or self-control with respect to food and drink

You are apathetic with respect to your physical condition.... You don't give a damn.

Chapter Thirteen

THE
COMPETITIVENESS
FACTOR

THIS WAS ONE OF THE MOST difficult chapters for me to write. I am aware that for very, very, many individuals competition can be a great thing. Competition can almost be a way of life for some individuals. For some individuals, competition has driven them to amazing accomplishments. But focusing on competition can be a great thing and can also be a substantial detriment to an individual's involvement in sports or other activities where there is some type of performance measurement or standard or comparison with others. Or simply, where there are winners and losers or where an event is timed (track, swimming etc) or measured (weight lifting, contests at work, etc.). How is this relevant to being fat or physically being out of shape? Well, quite obviously, the more active an individual the more likely said individual is not an Overly Fat Person. So first, let's take the negatives of competitiveness.

NEGATIVES OF COMPETION

I was very fortunate growing up. I attended a small Grade School and then a small High School. It was fortunate for me with respect to the competitive aspects of life but not so great with others. I was never the fastest. I was never the strongest or never the most agile. But because of the small genetic sampling in my sparsely populated town, I was able to be most certainly "average" or slightly above average in many areas. This may not have been the case if I had attended a large High School in a large metropolitan area with thousands of students.

Why is this important you ask? Well, think back on games played in grade school. Tag, Dodge Ball, informal sandlot football games, games in P.E. class etc. How soon do you think it took the individual who was always "it" in tag to realize he or she would never be a track star or a running back in High School let alone in High School, College or the NFL? How long did it take some individuals playing a Dodge Ball game to realize that they could not throw the ball as fast as others even if they practically threw their arm out? These individuals knew pretty darn fast. How do you think this made these kids feel with regard to sports, their peers, and their self-respect? How do you think this affected how they pursued/approached their later years with respect to activities, sports, etc.? Do you think it was positive? Add this realization to the constant "you can be anything you want to be or do anything you want if you try hard enough" and you have another reason for individuals to feel discouraged and ultimately cease participation in a multitude of activities.

Now, let's move on to High School (a period in my life I would just as soon forget). Let's also add the increased emphasis on competition, winning, and what bothers me the most, what I previously mentioned, " If you want it bad enough you can be anything you want in life." Now I should point out that part of this discussion is also reiterated in the "Genetics" chapter (and NO, mentioning genetics does not contradict my views). But the focus here is how does this emphasis on winning and performing well affect young adult lives with respect to activities they enjoy and pursue as adults.

For me, and like I stated earlier, I was fortunate to have gone to a small High School and it wasn't so terrible with respect to competition. I was able to compete somewhat in both team and individual sports and performed adequately. In track I was able to run in District Meets and even a State Track Meet. But what if I had attended a large High School? With the times I ran I may have barely made the track team let alone have been able to compete in District or State meets. What would this have done to me mentally and socially? How would it have affected my adult pursuits with respect to physical activity? Would it have made sports fun and something I wanted to continue later in life? Or would it have made sports something I dreaded, something that maybe I only did to "fit in" with my peers?

Most of my adult life I have been very active. I have enjoyed very much running, both sprinting and middle and long distances (I have run sprints in State Games scenarios and I have also completed a marathon) I have played competitive tennis, and have 3 years of martial arts experience. I weight lift and when heavily into lifting have been able to bench 23 reps of the NFL combine weight, which is 225lbs. But if I had gone to a large High School with many good athletes would I have continued to run or have enjoyed running so much? I doubt it. Would I have, if not for a Community College opportunity, spent many a day and hours on the tennis court? Probably not.

So the important aspect of this is what would I have done for physical activity as an adult if I had been in an environment when I was young where I was not even close to being competitive? An environment when I was young where I was often humiliated by my performance based against others? How would I have stayed in shape then? And most importantly, how would I stay in shape as an adult?

And let's go back to the other item I mentioned that goes along with all this competitiveness B.S. The philosophy that, "you can be anything you want to be if you try hard enough." Now that is not true and I believe it at worst destroys lives and at the least discourages individuals from continuing certain activities.

You **can't** be anything you want to be. Are they (the proponents of this be anything you want to be…) saying that if I just ran more sprints and weight lifting more as a youth… and of course, "really WANTED it," that I would be a world-class sprinter? Are they saying that if I had just ran more miles and really "WANTED IT" that I would be a world-class marathon runner? Or if I had thrown more baseballs as a youth I would have had a 90 plus mph fastball? Yeah, right!

Like more examples that are not sports related? What if my parents had a piano in the house and done the proper infant learning exercises and musical lessons? Does that mean I would have composed symphonies before the age of ten like Mozart? Or, if I had played enough chess as a youth and been trained properly I would have been the next Bobby Fischer or other child chess prodigy? Of course not!

Yet we constantly tell our youth and students this bullshit. And how does it make many feel. Well, I dare to say it sure makes the track athlete who trains twice as hard as the star runner feel like shit. But I know, we are trying to encourage our youth to pursue their dreams. To "be all they can be." Well, that's just all fine and dandy if we communicate to our youth that everyone **has his or her own strengths and weaknesses.** It would also be fine and dandy if we made sure that we communicate that not everyone can be a track star or a NBA athlete; that not everyone can be analytical or intelligent enough to be a nuclear physicist or a computer programmer. But we don't!

All these examples of telling our youth or even adults that they can be anything they want if they just put forth enough effort and the emphasis on competition causes people at an early age or as adults to avoid activities that they may enjoy or wish to participate just because they can't perform at a certain level and thus feel inadequate.

Now lets revert back to competitiveness with others. How many people stop jogging because when they tell people they run 10 minute miles they are laughed at by others.

How many people stop working out at the fitness center because they feel foolish when some roided out dude bench-pressing right beside them is doing reps with 3 times the weight?

So you ask, how does all of this relate to people being disgustingly fat? This relates to obesity because all of this disillusionment due to competitiveness with others or still having the thought process that endorsees that you can be anything you want if you just try hard enough leads to inactivity. Inactivity does not burn calories; activity burns calories. Not only does activity burn calories but also if you are doing something active there is a high likelihood that you are not simultaneously doing something to create obesity. Such as stuffing your face full of food! This is killing two birds with one stone. You are burning calories and taking in fewer calories. But this is not happening if you are disillusioned by competition.

CLUB OR HOME?

One-way of avoiding competition destroying your self-esteem and motivation is to avoid scenarios that put a great emphasis on competition. Yes, I know, that is pretty obvious isn't it! But some examples are not as obvious as it might appear. Let's take for example the fitness center.

You can probably see where this is headed. With competition being so bad for so many why do so many subject himself or herself to the feeling of inadequacy by going to fitness clubs instead of working out at home? How do you think the fitness clubs make money and yet don't have fitness centers totally overflowing with people? They have memberships available and room in their fitness centers because people drop out. Why? There are many reasons why people drop out of fitness centers and sport clubs. Some people are just plain lazy with no self-discipline to force themselves into working out and end up dropping their membership. Some people "over do it" initially and burn themselves out because they are competing with others, whether they know it or not. Some women quit after seeing the petite gorgeous blond on the Stairmaster and thinking to themselves, "I can never be like that." Or a man or a woman could be embarrassed about their appearance and quit due to being overly self-conscious. Guys can see the roided out dude benching ungodly amounts of weight and think, "why bother?" "I can never be like that guy." Still other people quit the clubs because of the time factor involved. Driving to the club, changing, working out, showering, and driving to work or back home; it just takes up too much of the day; with commitments at home and at work it is just not feasible.

So what did the previous paragraph make you think? Really, should a person workout at home or in a fitness center? Conversely, why should someone go to a fitness center? For one, there is the socialization factor. And although this may contribute to less of a workout for some, the competition and impression factor (Impressing peers) may increase workout loads for others. And of course, relating to the socialization factor, is the Male –Female thing. Nothing can make a guy squeeze out additional reps like a cute girl working out nearby. Of course this can be distracting as well. It can also cause injuries! And of course, there is the competition. And if it is the competition that drives you on, then by all means continue! But for many the fitness center is a dead end!

So why go through this? You shouldn't go through this. What should a person do? Just start working-out at home.

At home you can work out at your own pace. You are competing with yourself not people with different genetic characteristics. You have eliminated any travel/commute to the fitness center.

The fitness center is just one example of how people that should probably avoid competition can still workout and how avoiding the competition is beneficial for them. The same philosophy can be taken with running (avoid the tracks and races), tennis (play at lower levels of proficiency and or avoid tournaments) golf, etc.

POSITIVES WITH RESPECT TO COMPETION

THERE ARE DEFINITELY POSITIVES TO COMPETITION. Competition, democracy and freedom are what have made our nation great! Competition in sports brings athletes to new heights of accomplishments. Competition in business is Capitalism and most in our great nation still feel this is a great thing (excepting of course the President). So let's briefly go into why competition is great for certain individuals with respect to their fitness and weight control and also discuss two types of competition.

COMPETTION WITH YOURSELF

SO WHAT IS THE BEST TYPE of competition? From my perspective for the majority of the population I strongly feel the best type of competition is competition with yourself. The plus side of competition with yourself is that you will have a greater likelihood of not becoming depressed by your performance in any activity in relation to others, thus continuing this loved activity for an extend period of your life. The down side is that without competitions against others many would not realize their full potential due to not actually attaining a 100% level of effort. And sorry folks, I don't buy into the 110% garbage. An individual can only put forth 100% and any future gains are due to improved training, strategy, etc. or realizing that you were not giving 100% initially. A good example of a person not realizing they are not giving 100% effort is to take the sport of running, especially middle or long distance running. Some runners are able to get more out of themselves after witnessing what other runners accomplish or simply doing better by having other runners "pull" them along. But running is rather unique in that to push yourself 100% feels a little like trying to kill yourself, and competing against others basically just gets a person over the mental barriers of what is possible without grave physiological consequences (uhmm, like death).

But to me the pluses outweigh the negatives if you compete against yourself. I know personally that if I compared my running times with that of many other runners I would have given up running long ago due to depression or embarrassment. I vividly remember one year when I ran in the State Games of Oregon in the 35 or 40 year old age division. I was, for me, in extremely good overall condition. I was actually feeling great with my track workouts running great trial times (for me) and finishing pretty strenuous interval workouts on the track feeling pretty strong. So then I ran the 200 meters in the State Games and some guy beat me by about 10 yards (For you non-track people, 10 yards in a sprint is a mile!). My time was actually pretty decent for me as I was only off by only a few tenths of a second from my best time trial of that summer. But guess what? Even though I told myself to only be concerned with my own time and not that of others, what do you think happened? Well, I became depressed as hell. Suddenly I was asking myself, "Why on earth do I even bother running?" Suddenly, instead of feeling great about my physical condition I was depressed. Suddenly, going out the door for my maintenance runs was a chore and no longer enjoyable. Because of what? Because of, whether conscious or not, I was comparing myself with others who either trained harder or had more genetic running ability.

So now, when feeling competitive, I just time myself on the track or on a run to gauge my progress. With respect to weightlifting, I just compare what I have done in the past with respect to reps, weight and my body weight and use those measurements as a standard. And I know, you mental monsters and genetically gifted individuals are probably laughing at me now, but having my existing attitude of competing only against my previous performances allows me to continue to enjoy running, weightlifting, etc. And I guarantee all you readers (hopefully plural) that there are many people who have had similar experiences such as mine. And I am sure many of these negative experiences suffered by individuals have left them disenchanted with a previously loved activity or sport. And this disenchantment all because they didn't just compete against themselves or others of like abilities.

Another aspect of competition that needs analysis deals with the intensity of a persons training, whether through self-competition or competition against others. There are basically two ways to look at this intensity level issue. One, an individual should use all his or her intensity while they have the motivation to be intense, thus losing as much weight as possible quickly as possible. The second thought is to train at an intensity level with which an individual feels comfortable and can maintain this intensity for the long haul. And of course there could be strategies of a combination of the intensities such as training intensely initially with a plan to taper off after a certain period of time.

As one can easily see there are pluses and minuses to either approach with respect to training/workout intensity. Obviously, if you train very intensely initially, you run the risk of burning yourself out. This can be mental burn out or physical fatigue that could remain for extended periods of time. This can be especially true if an individuals training is coupled with an intense diet that is severely limiting caloric intake. The danger of the likelihood of burnout is real (think about the health clubs never being full membership wise) and can severely affect an individual's long-term goal of physical fitness and weight loss. On the other hand, gee…when an individual is motivated, go for it! Take advantage of this motivation, lose as much weight as possible and get fit as possible and then taper off when the onset of burnout raises its ugly head.

What is the authors view on this subject of workout intensity with respect to fitness and losing weight? What is my personal strategy and what strategy do I feel is best for others? With respect to my personal strategy, in the past, in my youth I was all for the training as intensely as possible for as long as possible. As I have aged, my view has changed significantly. My goal and philosophy with respect to fitness is, "Least amount of effort, for the maximum amount of gain." My philosophy deals with the law of "diminishing returns." If a person trains for one hour they will lose weight at a certain rate and will increase fitness level at a certain rate. But if this same individual doubles his or her training and trains for two hours a day, his or her weight loss and fitness level will most likely **not** double.

In addition, the doubling of the training load will definitely increase the likelihood of burnout and injury. For the average American, my strategy is somewhat similar to the "least amount of effort" philosophy. I feel for the average person, especially the non-athlete, having less intense workouts or activities and focusing more on an intense diet is the best method. For one, it is a hell of a lot easier to not intake an additional 500 hundred calories than it is to burn off 500 calories. Another factor is that when dieting energy levels will be lower thus making intense workouts much more difficult mentally and physically and for the average individual this will more then likely lead to burnout and the cessation of both the diet and exercise/activity.

COMPETITION AGAINST OTHERS

COMPETITION AGAINST OTHERS CAN BE GREAT for many individuals. If you are a competitive individual this competition against others can create intense internal motivation and determination and lead to vast improvements with respect to physical fitness and or weight control. For those individuals who are competitive and are by chance reading this book there is probably not a lot I can mention or suggest that they don't already know. If you are a competitive individual you probably already belong to that basketball or baseball league. If you are competitive and are a runner you probably already compete in the road races or track meets and more than likely know many methods of training. I could go on and on with examples but I believe I have made my point.

However, for those of you who need or would like more insight, another thought that comes to mind with respect to competitiveness is that some people are competitive with respect to activities that don't aid in weight control or physical fitness. I feel that these competitive individuals might try to channel that competitive energy toward an activity that involves some form of physicality. This would aid them greatly with respect to fitness levels and weight control. However, it is also entirely possible that maybe these competitive individuals don't participate in physical activities and sports because they are not proficient in these activities and because of their competitiveness, engaging in these activities and not achieving a high level of success is not an option. To these individuals, I suggest the already previous suggestion of just competing against oneself, thus avoiding what is for them the disgrace of not excelling.

Lastly, I guess the only point that needs reiteration with respect to competition against others and people who are extremely competitive is not to let the competitiveness become all-consuming. Don't let your competitiveness negatively impact your life with respect to your family, career, or other areas of importance. But a little bird tells me that if you are an Overly Fat Person that being so competitive and having the self-discipline to train yourself relentlessly will not be a potential problem.

So, in conclusion, the degree of competitiveness that is beneficial for any one person achieving a good level of physical fitness and/or a significant weight loss is a very individual matter. As in all aspects of life an individual needs to determine what method works best for them; not what method is most highly recommended or works best for others. Determine a method that works for you with respect to fitness and weight control and have the self-discipline to maintain this over your lifetime and you will be a happy, healthy and content individual.

IF YOU ARE OVERWEIGHT...

YOU ARE NOT:

"PORTLY"

YOU ARE NOT:

"A BUNDLE OF LOVE"

YOU ARE NOT:

"PLUS SIZED INDIVIDUAL"

YOU ARE FAT!

CHANGE YOUR LIFESTYLE!

REMEMBER!!!!!!! IF YOU ARE FAT IT IS BECAUSE OF ONE OR MORE OF THE FOLLOWING:

You are lazy and inactive

You lack any discipline or self-control with respect to food and drink

You are apathetic with respect to your physical condition.... You don't give a damn.

Chapter Fourteen

SOCIETAL ACTIONS

WHAT SHOULD WE AS INDIVIDUALS AND society do with respect to our nations obesity problem? For the sake of simplicity I will divide the actions/solutions into two different categories. The first category is for those individuals and groups of society that are not obese. The second category, if you have not already guessed, is for those who are Overly Fat Persons.

NORMAL SOCEITY

THE FIRST CATEGORY, THE GROUP OF individuals and entities that are not obese, unfortunately, comprises the smallest portion of the population. The most important action and or attitude that this group can take is that of NOT "feeling sorry" for obese people. Feeling sorry for fat people only conditions them into believing there is little they can do about their condition and also tends to make these fat individuals feel sorry for themselves; or worse yet, it allows fat people to not only rationalize their sorry state but to believe they are normal and even beautiful and sexy (If you are one of the few who think grossly fat people are beautiful then you have probably not read this far in the book and I have really no words for you other then there are a lot of perverse fetishes out there today).

The second thing we as normal individuals can do to help rid our nation of this fat epidemic is to treat individuals who are obese justly. What is justly you ask? Well, if you believe that people are fat due to the three reasons I have been continually harping upon since the forward of this book, then you should not respect obese people as much as an individual who has maintained a normal, healthy and good looking body. Why should you respect someone who has no self-control? Why should you respect someone who has no self-respect or dignity and lets themselves become fat slobs and not give a hoot!

For those who might be having difficulty accepting such attitudes (and I am sure there are many) it might be easier for you if you adopt a reverse attitudinal philosophy. If you can't bear to treat someone with disrespect who is obese then at least treat those of the population that maintain their fitness with increased respect.

A perfect example of treating those with more respect who HAVE self-discipline and dignity would come into play in the workplace. All you Hiring Managers and HR people out there; is not having self-discipline, motivation and dignity a great personality/character trait? If you are hiring a Salesperson for example, would you hire someone who is active and self-motivated, has self-discipline and keeps himself or herself in good shape or someone who is lazy, lacks self-discipline and has no respect for themselves?

Another factor that all Hiring Managers and HR employees should consider with relation to obesity and potential new hires is that of health. It is well documented both in this book and in millions of outside sources that being obese increases an individuals risk for many health related problems. So, and especially if your company offers and contributes to any portion of an employees health insurance, a Hiring Manager should be thinking of the "bottom line" with respect to the business at which they are working. In addition to increased health insurance premiums a business should be thinking of absenteeism in the workplace. If obese individuals have an increased risk for various health issues it stands to reason that it is more likely for an obese person to miss time at work.

Now I know many of you are thinking this is unfair. But why do you think this is unfair and possibly discrimination? Are not those characteristics mentioned with respect to one who stays in shape admirable qualities? Are they not qualities that typically exemplify top performing employees? So why not take these qualities into account? And thus, why not take fat people for what they are: lazy, lacking self-discipline and self-respect. Just remember, a person can't do anything with respect to their natural facial features (other than going under the knife) but a person does have control over their condition of obesity. So you Hiring Managers and HR staff, when a person arrives for an interview it is permissible to notice if they are obese; just as permissible as it is to ask about their self-motivation, discipline and pride.

What will the above-mentioned actions accomplish with respect to our nations obesity epidemic? Well, for one thing, if our society and individuals with power in the work place start treating Overly Fat People with some disrespect due to their lack of self-control and dignity, Overly Fat People will begin to realize that they must "get their act together" and lose some weight.

So why is this selection process not being implemented in our societies work place? Because there are the "fat sympathizers" and also the Overly Fat People themselves, who support those who are obese. Show me a 300-pound Hiring Manager and I'll show you a company that has many obese employees. Show me a Hiring Manager who is normal or in shape and I'll show you a company that has much less in the way of fat people. We all know, "birds of a feather flock together" and we know that "misery enjoys company." So there you have it; **this camaraderie amongst the fat is one reason why and how the obese survive.**

HELPING THOSE WHO ARE OVERWEIGHT

I KNOW, I KNOW, FOR MOST of this book I have been highly critical of those who are overweight and this, in my opinion, is totally justifiable. But having been slightly overweight at various times of my life I can see many of the obstacles that people who are presently overweight face. So I would like to offer some encouraging words to those who are Overly Fat People.

I think one of the biggest obstacles that face obese individuals might be that of HOPELESSNESS. I feel this sense of hopelessness, of feeling getting fit is a lost cause, may be prevalent amongst obese individuals. I feel this way because even though I have never been obese, I have been about 15 or so pounds overweight, and know the difficulty in just losing that much weight. So it is not extremely difficult for me to empathize, to place myself in the shoes of a severely obese person, and realize that this person may perceive their situation of having to lose as much as 100 pounds or more, as hopeless. It is especially easy to empathize the difficulty of an obese person has when faced with losing weight when I consider that I was only about 15 pounds overweight but I was physically fit enough to be able to not only limit my caloric intake but I was capable of exercising strenuously. Many obese people don't have this luxury of being able to exercise strenuously do to health consequences, physical limitations or other issues.

With this being said, what can we do to help those obese individuals who feel hopeless about their condition? It is readily obvious what these obese people need to do: that is overcome their laziness, lack of self-discipline and or apathy. But what can we do as a society to help the obese?

It is readily apparent that the present strategies of attempting to remedy our nations obesity problem have failed miserably. All the shortcut diets, foods, and supposedly unique exercise programs are at best only short-term solutions. Obviously, lifetime lifestyle changes must be made for obese people to permanently remain normal and healthy but if these obese people feel hopeless with respect to their condition they are extremely vulnerable to the quick fixes. And it is also obvious that our societies philosophy of basically condoning obesity and making obese people feel normal is no solution what so ever. So how can we help these people? What can our society offer to these obese individuals?

For one, people within our society who are normal can befriend those who are obese. You know the expression, "Birds of a feather flock together." Well, this is very true. So you individuals who are not fat make some friends with obese people and subtly encourage them to follow your examples. Make sure you are strong willed because the last thing you want is to start picking up the obese persons eating habits and lifestyle. So let obese people see how much you eat. Let obese people partake in your activities. Get your new obese friends up and moving and thinking about something other than what is for lunch. If you are a runner/jogger offer to go jogging with an obese person who may feel uncomfortable jogging alone. The same can be said with respect to any physical activity. An obese individual may feel extremely self-conscious at a gym if working out alone, so go with them to the gym. Or go for walks, play tennis, basketball, etc. with an Overly Fat Person. And above all offer words of encouragement to those who really do face an uphill battle after years of an unhealthy lifestyle.

But it is of vital importance NOT to encourage or condone obese individuals mindset that it is normal to be obese or that obesity is out of their control. This is what much of society does today and look where it has taken us. It has led us to a national epidemic of obesity.

THE OBESE

THIS, IN A ROUND (NO PUN intended) about way, now leads us to the second category of how we as a society should battle the nations obesity epidemic, and that relates to the obese people themselves. What can overweight individuals do to defeat this fat epidemic that threatens to destroy them and our nation? First, any fat person, just like any person who has a problem, must admit to himself or herself that they have a problem. Without this first step nothing of consequence can occur. If a fat person has just resigned themselves to being fat due to supposed genetic factors or just due to apathy, a remedy is not easily reached. Or if an Overly Fat Person believes the garbage with respect to "Big and Beautiful" or that it is natural for them to be fat, a remedy is also difficult to attain. But for those fat individuals who realize they have an issue and want to change their lives for the better it is strictly a matter of self-discipline. It is strictly a matter of individual accountability for ones own actions. **Get on that lifeboat!**

So if you're obese the rest is up to you. You have basically two paths of which to follow. The choice is yours. The important thing to remember is that you do have a choice and you can do something with respect to your obesity. So do it!

In summing up this chapter the important thing to remember is as a society it is of extreme importance not to, whether conscious or not, condone the physical state of obesity in others. This lack of accountability by obese individuals and societies empathy with these obese individuals is what has caused our nations obesity epidemic in the first place.

IF YOU ARE OVERWEIGHT...

YOU ARE NOT:

"AT RISK"

YOU ARE NOT:

"BIG AND BEAUTIFUL"

YOU ARE NOT:

"PLUMP"

YOU ARE FAT!

THINK OF YOUR FUTURE AND YOUR FAMILY!

REMEMBER !!!!!!!   IF YOU ARE FAT IT IS BECAUSE OF ONE OR MORE OF THE FOLLOWING:

You are lazy and inactive

You lack any discipline or self-control with respect to food and drink

You are apathetic with respect to your physical condition.... You don't give a damn.

Chapter Fifteen

THE OUTCRY

LIKE I MENTIONED IN THE FORWARD, this book threatens many. Any book that actually points out the facts and dispels many, many misleading theories on any subject will be met with skepticism, criticism, and even rage. Any book that could cost industries millions and millions of dollars will be met with intense resistance. Any book that threatens the unhealthy rationalization of fat people that their condition is uncontrollable will be trivialized or condemned. It is extremely important that this is mentioned and the reasons for these negative reactions be explored because a vast majority of the population and various interest groups will reject my book and theories whole-heartedly and with a passion reserved for life and death circumstances. So let's now explore some of the groups that will reject my book and the reasons why.

FAT PEOPLE

THE FIRST GROUP THAT WILL LIKELY reject my book will be the OFP's/Overly Fat People. Not all Overly Fat People mind you, but many. Congratulations to the Overly Fat People that don't reject this book because if this book is taken to heart these fat people will be on the way to a better life. But those that reject the book will do so for various reasons.

OFP's will not like the fact the author is showing society, and rightly so, that they are disgustingly fat and the accountability is theirs. They, the fat people, prefer to live their life rationalizing that they are fat for hundreds of reasons. And of course all these reasons are supposedly out of their control (hogwash). The fat population just doesn't want to face facts. The fat population wants no accountability for their actions. And they also **like** the fact that presently a large portion of the normal/non-fat population no longer calls them names or looks at them with disgust, either because it would not be politically correct or because they sympathize with the fat condition of these individuals. Believing in the writings in this book would change all that. They, the fat people, would hate the fact that this book reveals their true personality to the rest of society; that fat people are lazy, have no self-control, or just don't give a rat's ass. Gee, obese individuals might actually have to get off their fat asses and do something to alter the repulsive body that is theirs. They might actually have to use some self-control at the dinner table! Terrible! How terrible! This group of fat people, on the whole, will hate this book.

FAT SYMPATHIZERS

THE SECOND GROUP OF INDIVIDUALS OR entities, which will condemn this book, will be the "Fat Sympathizers." This group of Fat Sympathizers feels empathy toward the fat people in our society for various reasons. One of the reasons the Fat Sympathizers feel empathy toward fat people is because they feel these peoples obesity is out of their control (disease, mental condition/eating disorder, etc.). Another common belief among these Fat Sympathizers is that it is a natural condition for persons to be fat due to things such as genetics, aging, etc.

So seeing the Fat Sympathizers feel the reasons most people who are fat is out of their control they may then feel I am being unjustly critical of a fat person. They will feel that this book humiliates Overly Fat People. Some of these Sympathizers will feel that my views constitute a bias/discriminatory attitude toward fat people and this will be harmful in our society.

But of course my view is that for the past 30 years or so our society has been much too lenient and much too sympathetic toward Overly Fat People and this is a major contributing factor with respect to our nations fat epidemic. But hey, why should people be held accountable for their actions? Right? Geezz!

THOSE THAT WOULD LOSE

ANOTHER GROUP OR GROUPS THAT WILL hate this book will be those that stand to lose massive amounts of revenue. Let's take a look at some of the entities that stand to lose much in the way of revenue if people were to take the philosophies of this book to heart.

FOOD BASED DIET PROGRAMS

WITHOUT NAMING NAMES; AND I DON'T think it is at all necessary; I think it is obvious the organizations to which I am referring; the organizations that provide the actual food to which one is supposed to consume when on their diet plan. Don't get me wrong, these plans often times work. My objection to them is that they are ripping off the naïve consumer of thousands and thousands of dollars of hard earned money. And there is no need for the consumers to be spending hundreds of dollars each month on the programs food.

Why is this the case? If you take a quick glance at the food/nutritional information on these meals that are provided on these diet plans and one thing will really stand out. Each meal, although possibly very tasty and fantastic in appearance (I don't know if they taste good, I haven't wasted my money on them), has one characteristic. Each meal is low in calories! Amazing! To think that you can actually lose weight by the intake of less calories! What a novel concept; that you can actually lose weight by reducing your caloric intake! Gee, maybe if you had half a brain you would be capable of just eating less food. Purchase the food at a grocery store in bulk and you save money, have the variety you choose and not feel tied to a program. But of course you won't just buy less food you will try one of these programs due to the magnificent marketing campaign put forth by these entities. For instance, these entities tell you it is not the reduced calories that help you lose weight, it is the scientifically formulated recipe that combines just the right amount of carbohydrates, protein, etc. that make the pounds come off. Yeah, right!

Yes, you very well could lose much weight using these special food programs. But ultimately you will want to stop spending money on these programs and purchase food at everyday type locations such as grocery stores, restaurants, etc. But like I have emphasized in this book, a lifestyle change as far as eating habits and probably physical activity, is in order. If you lose the weight with one of these programs that provides meals, once you stop purchasing and consuming these meals if you revert back to your old eating habits you will gain back the weight. And what will you think about your weight gain? "Oh, I must not be eating the right balance of specialized carbohydrates and protein." Jeeeezzzzz. Why not change your eating habits up front, become accustomed to selecting and purchasing your own meals at your local grocery store, and not have some difficult transitional period after discontinuing the Diet/Meal type program? Of course, if you want to provide these companies with a steady revenue source go right ahead. **Maybe you should also purchase their stock!**

So the bottom line is these companies will hate this book because of possible revenue loss if the Overly Fat People in our society who are trying to lose weight discontinued or never start purchasing their products and just ate less of what they are already eating.

DIET PILL AND SUPPLEMENT MFG'S

IF ALL YOU DO IS JUST simply lower your caloric intake and follow basic principles in this book, or really any sound advice from a nutritionist, then another group of companies stand to lose money. These are the companies that manufacture and sell diet pills. Whether the pills are to suppress an individual's appetite or if they are designed to increase one's metabolism or both, these companies will hate this book and the ideas expressed within.

The problems I have with these pills/drugs are maybe not as many as you might imagine. My main concerns with the various types of diet pills on the market are the effectiveness of the pills, the health effects on an individual's body and whether a person will become dependent on the pills.

EFFECTIVENESS

WITH RESPECT TO THE EFFECTIVENESS OF the pills I have not done massive amounts of research. Much of my opinion is based on having in the past actually trying some of these so-called wonder diet pills. The other opinions I have regarding these pills is based on the disclaimer that the FDA has not determined if the claims of these pill manufacturers products are legit.

Gee, could these companies just be playing on the fact that fat people in our society just want a quick solution to their obesity problem and are gullible enough to spend their money for these pills? No, that couldn't be! Could it?

And of course these diet pill companies have great marketing and advertising campaigns. "Are you under stress? Are you over weight in the abdomen, hips and thighs?" "Then you need ABC diet pills." Hey, what kind of idiot would fall for such blatant propaganda buy this "sucker," type advertising? MILLIONS. But hey, you're under stress, right? You have gained weight in the areas mentioned, right? Then what they're saying must be correct, right? Besides, the models they use look thin, right? It's on T.V. or the Internet so it must be true, right? **Hey guys and girls, what turnip truck have you just fallen off?**

But what the heck. If you have or are trying any of these pills and they are working for you keep right on taking them. I mean, the placebo effect is scientifically proven. But seriously, some of the products do aid in the reduction of a persons weight and I really have no problem with the proven products. If a certain product helps a person lose weight that is great! **I just wish fat individuals in our society had more discipline and would lose weight just by self-control and not needlessly make these entities wealthy by consuming their products.**

DEPENDENCE AND EFFECT AFTER DISCONTINUATION

IF THE PILLS OR DRUGS HAVE worked for you, well then that's great (I am actually being serious now). There is however one big potential problem. And that problem begins once you stop taking the drugs. Of course you could eliminate this problem by taking these drugs the rest of your life. But I don't think most people consider this an option.

So what happens now that you stopped taking the drugs? If they are based on appetite suppression you have been eating less and this affect will probably last for a while. You may or may not have developed a better sense of the difference between hunger and cravings or emotional needs. But after awhile there is a very good chance you will revert back to your old eating habits. Then what? What do you think.................You will again purchase these pills from manufactures and start the cycle all over again.

If the drugs were metabolism based what do you think happens when you stop. Well, you might be in luck if because of the pills increasing your metabolism you increased your daily activities due to your increased energy levels. Maybe these habits... if they are now indeed habits, will continue forward. But in all likelihood they will not. Then what happens? What do you think? More money out of your pocket!

So, the diet/supplement industry will hate this book because I promote people losing weight by more natural means and thus saving the dieter money in both the long and short term. And this conversely will lower the revenues of many companies thus causing these entities to very much dislike philosophies put forth in this book.

EXERCISE PROGRAMS AND DEVICES

THE EXERCISE PROGRAM AND EXERCISE MACHINE/IMPLEMENTS/ DEVICES entities are another group of entities that stand to lose much revenue. If fat people would just cut calories and engage in simple physical activities when wishing to lose weight or maintain physical fitness many of these entities that produce or promote ways to lose weight would lose money. And thus, these entities are diametrically opposed to simple and natural methods to lose weight or stay fit and will hate this book. The biggest problem with most of these devices or programs is that they promise the world to people who's thoughts are well meaning, that of losing weight and getting fit, but are extremely susceptible to people or companies promising the moon, earth and sky (or however that old expression goes). Just like people wanting financial independence are susceptible to money scams promising riches, or unemployed individuals gullible to the promises of potential employers or multi-level marketing plans, many fat people actually want to lose weight, look and feel better, but are victims waiting to be had for the unscrupulous company wanting to sell their goods and products that supposedly make losing weight easy.

*I guess I should point out that I am a firm believer (if you haven't figured it out yet) in activity and exercise. I am not being critical of tried and true fitness machines or exercise programs. My disgust is aimed more at the companies that, for instance, advertise an Abs Machine and claim you will lose massive amounts of weight by using their machine 5 minutes a day 3 times a week and doing **nothing else**. What a joke!*

Our nations public, although intelligent, is also extremely gullible. People will believe almost anyone who has supposed authority, anyone with a white doctors coat or named Milgram. Or for that matter, the public will believe and trust anyone who promises utopia, is handsome and reads well from a teleprompter. It somehow is not significant to the gullible public that said individual attends a racist church, associates with unrepentant terrorists, and surrounds himself with self proclaimed communists, and for icing on the cake, tells us with disrespect that we should go cling to our Bibles and guns (I apologize for using this example twice and for becoming political, I was just trying to make a point). This same gullibility is a partial reason so many fat people try the diet pills or plans, the special foods, the special supposedly unique exercise programs, etc.

The other reason fat people try the food and pills and easy exercise programs that promise miracles are that many individuals are either lazy or just want the "quick fix." If an abdominal machine advertisement promises "5 minutes a day three times a week and you will lose inches" and the advertisement has a beautiful or handsome model using the machine then it "must be true," right?

This last example of the abdominal machine and the promises of quickly losing inches also leads to another problem of our society which I covered somewhat in other parts of this book; the problem of ignorance. Please take note of the word "ignorance" which was used instead of "stupidity." Some people in our age of enlightenment still are ignorant to basic physiological facts. Much of this ignorance is due to people seeing a 10 minute infomercial or reading a few short articles in magazines or reading some blogs on the internet and then believing they are knowledgeable with respect to physiology, exercise principles, etc.

One could rightfully argue that this "ignorance" in many individuals is not lack of knowledge but misinformation or propaganda put forth by money making entities. I tend to believe it is the influence of propaganda by the entities literally stealing millions from consumers as opposed to ignorance by the consumer. But I guess it comes down to whether you believe in the expression "Buyer Beware." Should the buyer be obligated to be somewhat informed? Should the buyer be protected by consumer groups... or the author? How much accountability should be placed with the consumer? Questions for the ages!

Again, the bottom line is these entities selling the exercise programs or machines would lose countless dollars if people attempting to lose weight used some logic and common sense with their approach to weight reduction. But, if I were a betting man, I would still invest in these entities stocks. Americans just won't learn.

ANTI-DIETING/ EATING DISORDER GROUPS

THERE IS YET ANOTHER GROUP OUT there in our society that will more then likely object to this book; that entity is the Eating Disorder Groups. The problem with a large percentage of these groups, and the ones to which I am focusing my attention, is that they are focusing their attention on individuals who are in their opinion, too thin. These groups especially like to direct their attention toward Supermodels who in their opinion set a bad example for our society, especially young women. These groups are concerned that young women see these thin supermodels as role models and that in order to emulate the supermodels; young impressionable women will develop eating disorders, specifically Bulimia and Anorexia. These groups concerned with eating disorders will see this book as yet another problem for our youth, who in their estimation, are already inundated with too much in the way of propaganda to become or remain normal (oops, thin).

I will have to admit that I feel that someone who is relying on anorexia or bulimia to become so thin as to, in reality, be emancipated has a problem. But from purely visual evidence; evidence that is looking us right in the eye everyday, our society has a much more serious problem with obesity than with young emancipated women or women with eating disorders such as Bulimia. Ask yourself this the next time your at the shopping mall; do you see a lot of teenage girls who look too thin? Do you see teenage girls so thin and emancipated that you should notify the authorities because their parents must be neglecting them? Of course not! What you are more likely to witness at the mall is that of countless teenage girls who are fat. These OFP who are still young are in for a terrible life of weight and health issues. And in my opinion, these groups that are so worried about the health of our youth should focus on the obese population of our country and be concerned with these obese peoples health and the cost to our society.

Now I know, these groups concerned with eating disorders with respect to our youth wanting to be thin will counter with some argument such as, "We are concerned with the health of our youth and that too many girls are trying to be something they are not.... "Thin." These groups will insist that not everyone is meant to be thin and some of us are naturally fat. I counter with examples from my chapter on genetics such as the "lifeboat scenario" or inhabitants of 1942 Stalingrad or even the Donner Party (Yes, maybe the Donner Party did have an eating disorder). Were these individuals genetically predisposed to THINNESS???? Where were all the genetically prone fat people in these just mentioned examples?

Consider this article from OMG! This is a prime example of how certain groups fear our youth trying too hard to be thin. On Yahoo. com posted by Lindsay Robertson on Thursday November 19th 2009

> Dimitrios Kambouris/WireImage.com Groups representing the anti-eating-disorder movement in the U.K. are blasting supermodel Kate Moss for a seemingly offhand remark she made in a recent interview with the fashion website *WWD*. When asked about her personal motto, Moss said: "There are loads. There's 'Nothing tastes as good as skinny feels.' That's one of them. You try and remember, but it never works."

Now heaven forbid if people in the world are actually concerned with being fit! It must really bother all those lazy, undisciplined, apathetic fat people out there that other people care about their bodies. These groups of individuals who are actually concerned with their appearance and physical fitness must really bother them. Fit individuals make these eating disorder groups and fat people in general cognizant of the fact that they are overweight and not healthy; so they think, let's attack the fit and healthy, they make me feel uncomfortable!

In conclusion, there are many groups that will detest the views contained within these pages. The reasons are many, from loss of revenue, loss of the perceived view that individuals are not accountable and from the supposed political incorrectness that is presented.

IF YOU ARE OVERWEIGHT...

YOU ARE NOT:

"HEAVY"

YOU ARE NOT:

"FULL FIGURED"

YOU ARE NOT:

"CHUBBY"

YOU ARE FAT!

DON'T EAT SO DAMN MUCH!

REMEMBER!!!!!!! IF YOU ARE FAT IT IS BECAUSE OF ONE OR MORE OF THE FOLLOWING:

You are lazy and inactive

You lack any discipline or self-control with respect to food and drink

You are apathetic with respect to your physical condition.... You don't give a damn.

CONCLUSION

FIRST, I WOULD LIKE TO STATE that I appreciate anyone who has read this book. This appreciation stems not only from monetary reasons but because I believe that our nation is handling the obesity epidemic in an incorrect manner. And thus, if you have read my book up to this point, maybe, just maybe I have convinced you of our societies misguided attitudes toward obesity. I truly believe that a "tough love" and "accountability for ones actions" philosophy toward our nations obese individuals is the best possible solution to the obesity problem prevalent amongst not only the adult portion of our society, but sadly, also our youth.

In conclusion, this book has tried to dispel some myths with respect to losing weight. I have also discussed the propaganda that targets our nation and how it affects our populace. And I have also mentioned other related issues such as revenue seeking entities that take advantage of a fat persons desire of actually wanting to take action and become fit. I have stated that it is "calories in, calories out" and have given ample examples of why being obese is under an individuals control and how they can do something about their condition.

And remember, if you are obese and don't believe my concepts…

JUST JUMP ON THAT LIFEBOAT!!!!!!!!!!!!!!!

You will then become a believer!